CELEBR SMALL VICTORIES

My Journey Through Two Decades of AIDS Response

J.V.R. Prasada Rao

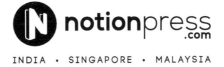

INDIA · SINGAPORE · MALAYSIA

Notion Press

No. 8, 3rd Cross Street
CIT Colony, Mylapore
Chennai, Tamil Nadu – 600004

First Published by Notion Press 2020
Copyright © J.V.R. Prasada Rao 2020
All Rights Reserved.

ISBN

Hardcase: 978-1-63714-553-1
Paperback: 978-1-63633-761-6

CONTENTS

FOREWORD

These pages trace the remarkable journey of a truly remarkable man. It is a real honour and an even greater pleasure to offer this foreword to the memoir of my long-time colleague and friend, J.V.R. Prasada Rao. Prasada has been at the forefront of the fight against HIV/AIDS at the national, regional, and global levels for more than two decades. I had the privilege of working closely with him in various capacities when I was the Executive Director of UNAIDS: from his time as the Director of the National AIDS Control Organisation in India, as Union Secretary for Health and Family Welfare of India, and the UNAIDS Regional Director for Asia and the Pacific, to his role as the United Nations Secretary-General's Special Envoy for AIDS in Asia and the Pacific.

I can think of few other people who have made such an indelible mark on the health and well-being of so many communities in India and around the world. This book is first and foremost about genuine leadership, enshrined in science and evidence (as a nuclear physicist by training), with a total dedication to serving people and communities. Throughout his long career, J.V.R Prasada Rao has combined wisdom with determination, and activism with political realism. He is just as at ease in international institutions as he is at the community level, and has always been committed to generating meaningful results for some of the most underserved communities in India and around the world.

Prasada is the architect of India's AIDS response. Among his many achievements, he played a pivotal role in implementing a comprehensive and decentralized national AIDS control programme in the country, thereby saving millions of lives. He is a rare example of a civil servant who can work directly with civil society to drive progress. For example, he has worked closely with sex workers, people who inject drugs, and the LGBTQ community to advance innovative solutions to address expressed needs in India and throughout the Asia Pacific region. From Bangkok to Mumbai, the book tells colourful and powerful stories about the importance of people-led action, community empowerment, and mutual learning.

I was particularly pleased to dive into Chapter 3 and reflect on the role of the extraordinary Independent Commission on AIDS in Asia Pacific, for which Prasada served as the Member Secretary. Dr. Chakravarthi Rangarajan, a renowned development economist and former Governor of the Reserve Bank of India, chaired the Commission, which looked at the unfolding realities of the HIV/AIDS epidemics in Asia. The Commission brought together an impressive multisector coalition of leading economists, scientists, civil society representatives, and policymakers from across the region. It was unique in taking a truly long-term view and looking beyond the health sector at the socioeconomic impacts of HIV infection. The Commission set out decisive actions for dealing with the acute HIV epidemics in Asia while planning for the future, and remains an exemplary model for tackling other health and societal issues around the world, as we are now seeing with the COVID-19 crisis as societies learn to live with the virus.

There are few people in the world who have combined such vast experience and broad perspective, and have done it with remarkable results. True to his character, Prasada tells it as it is throughout the book and we would all do well to heed the many lessons he shares.

We have made nothing short of spectacular progress in the AIDS response. It has been a collective effort and is a true success story. Yet with 1.7 million people newly infected with HIV in 2019 and nearly 700,000 deaths in the same year, the end of AIDS remains elusive. Prasada's book could not come at a more important time. The AIDS response is at a crossroads and, with it, the lives of millions of people are hanging in the balance. The sobering reality is that even before the COVID-19 crisis, we were not on track to end AIDS as a public health threat by 2030 and the COVID-19 pandemic risks shattering hard-won gains and reversing progress. The many lessons Prasada shares throughout his memoir–from the importance of political leadership and dedicated resources, broad coalitions and activism, to science and people-driven responses–will be essential in charting a path forward. It can be done but only if we counter prevailing complacency, take bold action, and stay united.

*– **Professor Peter Piot***
Director, the London School of Hygiene & Tropical Medicine,
and Former Executive Director, UNAIDS

PREFACE

In the public services sector, rarely does one get an opportunity for long and sustained engagement with an agenda of enormous global concern. In health sector no other public health issue has engaged the attention of the global community the way HIV/AIDS did in the past two decades, not just in the measure of devastation it had caused but also in the unprecedented response, driven by political commitment and financial support by countries and global agencies. I was fortunate to get the opportunity to not just observe this interplay, but also play a significant role in the global effort for two decades from 1997 to 2017.

In 1997, when I joined as Director of the National AIDS Control Organisation (NACO) in the Government of India, little did I realise that the AIDS epidemic in India was reaching its peak in prevalence and mortality. The country was still in a denial mode and support for a national effort to combat the epidemic was seriously lacking. For the next two decades I undertook the long and arduous journey of leading an intensified response in India, and later in the Asia Pacific region, rounding off my efforts in 2017 as the Special Envoy of the UN Secretary-General for AIDS. In these two decades, I enacted several roles–a leader, advocate, implementor and an activist in the global campaign to tame and halt the march of an epidemic which has consumed globally about 40 million lives and has another 30 million living with the virus. Strangely, at no stage of this sequence of events did I have any inkling that it will be so long and continuous without break.

I wanted this long sojourn to be recorded not as an exercise in epidemiology but as a personal narrative on an important societal issue with deep developmental implications, intertwining my responses, challenges, moments of triumph and despair with the unfolding of the epidemic in India and the rest of Asia Pacific. My effort has two objectives (1) to document and preserve the institutional memory from the formative years of the programme to serve as a guide for the future and (2) to inspire young aspirants of public health careers on how to confront major public health challenges while learning lessons from the past, and how they can become the harbingers of that change.

In this process I faced many challenges. I started working on this book in 2019 when my wife and I spent 4 months in California, United States, helping my son and daughter-in-law with their newborn baby girl. I had time to reflect on the events of the past 20 years, but the task of putting them in print was daunting. First, I am not a professional writer. There were many occasions in my career spanning over 40 years as a civil servant when I faced enormous work life challenges which could have filled pages of a few books. But all I did then was to do the job, move on and never look back. My writings were mostly limited to opinion pieces in newspapers on issues I felt compelling to write about.

In such moments one needs someone who can boost your confidence and push you to do those things which you consider impossible to accomplish. Such support came from unlikely quarters in the form of Sudhakar Kurapati. Sudhakar and I knew each other since my NACO days when he was working in USAID, one of the funding agencies of National AIDS Control Programme Phase II (NACP II). He moved to the World Bank and later to Centers for Disease Control and Prevention (CDC) technical team in India. We were in regular touch all these years. After completion of my tenure as Special Envoy of UN Secretary-General, Sudhakar started encouraging me to write down my experiences in the form of a book. It was not a casual suggestion but a persistent effort to convince me about the usefulness of such an effort. In early 2019, I finally decided to write this narrative.

I then wanted to sound out some colleagues I worked closely with before launching my effort. Prominent among them are Dr. Peter Piot, former UNAIDS chief and currently Director of London School of Hygiene and Tropical Medicine, London. He enthusiastically responded to my query with words of encouragement. Swarup Sarkar, my long-time friend and colleague also felt that it is important to document the efforts of the past two decades and helped me with important inputs.

As I started my work I could realise how difficult it was to recollect the past events of more than a decade and find proper references for my writings. In the 1990s, work in government was mostly carried out on paper and in files, and computers were just getting introduced in official work. E-mails were used only for interacting with external partners. I was not getting proper references about important landmarks in the national programme in India. There were occasions when I felt like abandoning the entire effort and going back to my normal routine. But the faces of those affected who I have met, their stories and suffering, which are now only part of a dusty document or an excel sheet somewhere gave me that additional impetus to give voice to their now silent suffering and capture them for posterity. I sounded out some more friends and associates who encouraged me and pledged their support. I could finally complete the manuscript after 18 months of arduous effort, ploughing through the information of the past 20 years and separating the grain from the chaff.

The book is titled *Celebrating Small Victories: My Journey Through Two Decades of AIDS Response* and captures important events and landmarks in the AIDS response with appropriate focus on my role in stimulating multisectoral involvement in formulating policies and scaling-up of programmes. The book essentially follows my journey since I, as mentioned in the prologue, started my first interaction with the National AIDS Control Programme in India. This initial exposure then deepens through chapters 1 and 2, elaborating my experiences from the time I joined NACO until my retirement as Secretary Health, Government of India (1997-2004). Chapter 3 outlines the regional response in Asia Pacific where I led the advocacy efforts as Director of the regional office of UNAIDS, the joint UN programme on AIDS in Bangkok from 2005 to 2009. Chapter 4 traces the events leading to the UN summit on Sustainable Development Goals in 2015 and my role as the Special Envoy of the UN Secretary-General in aligning countries to the global agenda of ending AIDS as a public health concern by 2030. Chapter 5 gives account of my work in the area of HIV and public health as a member of important civil society organisations in India and abroad. The narrative would end with an epilogue critically evaluating the current scenario of waning interest in AIDS control and contributory factors for this loss of focus at a crucial stage.

During this journey I was a witness to the devastation that AIDS caused in India and other countries of Asia Pacific to lives and livelihoods of people who were leading a precarious existence on the margins of society. More telling were the extreme levels of stigma and discrimination at work and in life that people had to suffer from mainstream society–even in the hands of health care providers. I had to plead with physicians and surgeons to provide these populations with even basic health care services to which they are normally entitled as citizens of a country. In premier institutions boards were displayed at the beds of AIDS patients disclosing their health condition–totally against the norms of privacy and confidentiality. In India, I had to fight objections from Planning Commission bureaucrats who tried to block the programme arguing against a focused national programme for AIDS and suggesting merger with health care system. On the positive side I met some extraordinary people who despite getting infected by HIV and without any treatment in sight were leading the civil society to fight against stigma and discrimination of HIV-positive persons. Many of them died at a young age but their battle to get antiretroviral (ARV) medicines into the national programme helped many others to survive.

A section of people I least expected to meet in my life were the key populations of sex workers, LGBTQ community and drug user populations. My introduction to these groups was an eye opener in terms of the crucial role they played in our societies even while remaining socially marginalised. The challenges they faced were unique, requiring innovative solutions. My initial introduction with them soon developed into a cordial and mutually beneficial relationship both in India and Asia Pacific region. It was not just the leaders but the foot soldiers of these communities who fought a valiant battle against social stigma and brought their communities into the centre stage of AIDS response. From the Thai AIDS orphan in Chiang Mai to the peer educator at Kamatipura in Mumbai, a whole new world unknown to many people unfolded before me in these two decades of work. These people were my inspiration for pushing me relentlessly to take up their cause in all available fora in India, in the Asia Pacific region and later at the global level. At the end, these experiences and the amazing people whom I met during this journey made me realise myself as a better human being.

As a side note, the ending of my efforts on this book dovetailed with the explosion of the Covid-19 epidemic onto the international scene and my own involvement, both at the state and national level in an advisory role. Although I was sorely tempted to shoehorn the Novel Coronavirus into this book and make it more topical, I decided to not give in. Although not without parallels, I was determined that the focus of the book should be on the AIDS challenge, for there is one thing that makes it unique. There is no vaccine, no cure, not even 40 years after it broke out into the open. Covid19 will find its way out of our daily conversation, after a cure and a vaccine are found in near future, but HIV in the current scenario will continue to reap a toll. It is a story that must be told, again and again, for each time we forget the lessons of the past, we come closer to a point of no return.

I struggled with the name of the book but the words of Peter Piot kept coming back to me again and again–in our fight with the virus we should not get disheartened but learn to celebrate small victories to move forward. The final victory is still eluding the world, but we must relentlessly move forward and celebrate these small and decisive victories on the way.

– *J.V.R. Prasada Rao*
Bangalore

ACKNOWLEDGEMENTS

This book would not have seen the light of the day without the direct and indirect contribution of many–family, friends, colleagues and well wishers. I gratefully acknowledge their great support by inspiring me, providing inputs and pumping me up whenever I wanted to give up.

My family beginning with my centenarian mother, my wife Usha and my two sons, Dinesh and Chandrasekhar, my daughter Sasi, their spouses and children were always with me in this venture and never allowed me to lose heart. In fact the entire project got unveiled when I and my wife visited the United States to spend a vacation with them in early 2019. They contantly encouraged me to tread the full path and reach the goal. My nephew, Rajeev, closely followed the progress of work and resolved many computer glitches that I encountered.

Peter Piot can't be thanked enough for being my inspiration during these two decades of my work on HIV/AIDS and even beyond. The sense of optimism which flows through the narrative is the result of the deep influence he had on my thinking and my work. The foreword he wrote for the book bears testimony to the value he ascribed to my work on HIV/AIDS for the past two decades.

C. Rangarajan, Pronab Dasgupta and Tom Frieden took pains to go through the draft and provided their incisive comments and suggestions which enriched the contents of the book.

I stated in the prologue how much I owe to Sudhakar Kurapati whose constant encouragement and support were most critical to turning my vision into reality. He provided valuable additions to the narrative which I would have otherwise missed.

Swarup Sarkar has been a cotraveller on my two decades of journey in Delhi, Bangkok and even later. He encouraged and constantly challenged me to do better.

Bhavna Yeshu Goyal undertook the onerous task to edit my manuscript. I briefed her over the phone what my book contains and she immediately agreed to take up the work. She understood all my fussiness about language, presentation and frequent changes in the narrative and carried out an excellent final draft of the book.

Many friends and former colleagues have encouraged me and provided vital inputs. Prominent among them were Pradeep Kakkattil, Mahesh Mahalingam, Salil Panakadan and Nandini Kapoor from UNAIDS, Tracy Newbury (formerly from RST UNAIDS), Tenu Avafia from UNDP New York, Salim Habayeb (formerly from the World Bank and WHO), Sanjeeva Kumar and Vinita Varma from NACO, Neelam Kapur and Mohammed Shaukat former colleagues from NACO, Bharat Rewari from WHO SEARO, G.V.S. Murthy from PHFI, Samiran Panda from ICMR, Anil Purohit from Jodhpur School of Public Health, Sunita Singh from Amaltas, Arif Jafar, Ashok Row Kavi, Elizabeth Selhore, Jahnabi Goswami, Mona Mishra, Smarajit Jana, Sundar Sundararaman and Vivek Anand from the civil society and key populations.

Watchareeporn Kulpisitthicharoen, my former executive secretary in RST Bangkok, refreshed my failing memory on many events relating to my work in the RST. She along with her colleagues, Prapapan Supreyaporn and Nisarat Wangchumtong helped me in accessing relevant parts of the archived material from my 5-year stay in Bangkok. The RST Data Hub is a storehouse of invaluable data and information on the regional AIDS response in Asia Pacific. Khin Cho and Ye Yu, the young Myanmarese technical staff, in the Hub rendered enormous help in accessing key published data about the epidemic from its website.

The voices of the communities infected and affected by HIV are the principal sources of inspiration for my decision to write on my two decades of journey combating the epidemic. I salute them for their courage and determination in carrying their fight for the right to a healthy and dignified life through all these turbulent years.

If writing this book is a daunting exercise, getting it printed and published proved to be an equally challenging task. I was a complete novice in this area. When I was all at sea struggling to get a good publisher on board, timely advice and support came from Anil Purohit, Deepanjan Sujit Roy and Bhavna Yeshu Goyal who identified Notion Press in Chennai for printing and publishing the book. The publisher presented an attractive cover design and an excellent publication as my first attempt at book writing.

APPRECIATION

Prasada Rao played a notable role in combating HIV/AIDS not only in India but also globally. From 1997 to 2017 he was deeply involved in formulating and implementing multiple programmes to prevent its spread. This interesting and challenging journey has been recorded in this book. The flow of the narrative is smooth and absorbing, and the book will remain as a good guide to experts and policy makers not only in HIV/AIDS but in all Public Health Programmes. For a public health programme to succeed there is the need for leadership, advocacy and activism. Prasada Rao possessed all these qualities in an abundant measure. Thus he was a soldier and general simultaneously. All these come through clearly, as one moves from one chapter to another of the book.

I came into contact with Prasada Rao when he met me with a request to Chair the Independent Commission on AIDS in Asia in 2005. Obviously, the membership of the Commission consisted of experts in different fields as well as activists and they were drawn from different countries. I saw at first-hand Prasada Rao's abilities in handling people with diverse backgrounds and the proceedings of the Commission went through smoothly largely because of him. The book tells about how the Report of the Commission was unique in many ways. In fact, the Commission had to decide given the limitation of the resources, the relative emphasis on prevention and treatment. We came to the conclusion that the most cost-effective approach would be to lay greater emphasis on prevention. However, the need for taking care of treatment could not be overlooked. If the report was a major landmark in the evolution of policies towards HIV/AIDS much of the credit must goes to Prasada Rao.

There are messages for all stakeholders in the fight against HIV/AIDS in the book. Prasada Rao's experience expanded from the national to the regional and finally to the global level. Part of his success as an administrator is his willingness to listen to others. In short, the book shows what an administrator with conviction and commitment can achieve and overcome challenges, however, formidable. The title of the book is *Celebrating Small Victories*. But small victories add up. As the proverb goes 'Little drops of water make the ocean mighty'.

– Dr. C. Rangarajan
Chairman, Madras School of Economics
Former Chairman, Economic Advisory Council to the Prime Minister of India
Former Governor, Reserve Bank of India

PROLOGUE

The mid-1990s were a period of transition in my career as a civil servant in India. For about a year from June 1996 to June 1997, I was serving as the Resident Commissioner of West Bengal Government in Delhi. The Commissioner is the resident representative of a state positioned in the national capital to maintain effective liaison between the state and the central governments. The representative manages an office and a Bhavan (like a guest house) in Delhi, which houses visiting state ministers and officials. It is a staid job in normal times but in times of political crisis it assumes huge importance because of the intricate and politically sensitive centre–state relations in India. My tenure coincided with such a critical period of political uncertainty when prime ministers of the country rotated in quick succession. The Chief Minister of West Bengal, Jyoti Basu from the Communist Party of India (Marxist), played a crucial role of kingmaker in some of these transitions involving two successive Prime Ministers, H.D. Deve Gowda and Inder Kumar Gujral.

As the dust was settling down on these political appointments, I along with my colleagues in the 1967 batch of Indian Administrative Service (IAS) were eagerly waiting for our elevation in rank and appointment as Additional Secretaries in the Government of India (GOI). The IAS is the premier civil service in India and its members are recruited through a tough all India entrance process conducted by the Union Public Service Commission of India. After working in rural sub-districts and districts, the officers hold senior management positions in the state governments they are allotted to after recruitment. They get the option of working in the GOI based on an empanelment process and move up the administrative hierarchy to occupy senior administrative positions such as secretaries in the GOI.

I was through with this empanelment process for appointment in the GOI and was waiting for appointment orders. On June 30, 1997, the GOI notified me as Additional Secretary in the Ministry of Health and Family Welfare and Project Director (PD) of National AIDS Control Organisation (NACO) established in 1992 for control of AIDS epidemic in India. I was happy that finally I was getting back to the GOI but the designation as PD NACO set me thinking. I heard about AIDS and HIV virus that causes this health condition; how it was spreading across the world and had become a public health challenge in India too. Beyond that I had no knowledge of its intensity and spread.

In India, the Ministry of Health and Family Welfare is a key constituent of national governance under Indian Constitution. Even though health figures in the list of subjects which fall under the mandate of state governments, the federal government has all the coordinating functions of setting policy, managing national programmes for disease control, organising health research and promoting public health. During my tenure it was divided into the following three departments:

1. The Department of Health dealing with most of the policy and regulatory aspects of health.
2. The Department of Family Welfare looking after population, reproductive and child health and development aspects of health.
3. The Department of Indigenous Systems of Medicine named as AYUSH, signifying Ayurvedic, Unani, Siddha and Homeopathy systems of medicine.

Each of these departments was headed by a secretary supported by senior officials of the rank of additional secretaries and joint secretaries. The Department of Health functioned as the coordination wing of the ministry.

The ministry provides substantial resources to the states for national programmes, which are classified as central sector projects and centrally sponsored schemes. The central sector projects are fully funded by the

GOI and centrally sponsored schemes are funded by both central and state governments in a predetermined ratio.

My role in this huge government setup was to support the health secretary in policy and budgetary matters and to administer important national programmes for disease control. The implementors of these programmes were technocrats in the Directorate General of Health Services (DGHS), which is the main technical wing of the health ministry. The exception was HIV/AIDS, where I was directly in charge of implementation of the national programme as Project Director (PD) NACO specially constituted for managing the national response. I would reserve for discussion in the next chapter on how AIDS was given this special status and how a separate organisation called NACO had to be constituted to administer the programme.

On 7 July 1997, when I went to assume charge in the health ministry headquarters in Nirman Bhavan, I realised that even before my joining I became the centre of a tussle between the Minister of State for Health (MoS) and the Health Secretary about allocation of my work in the Ministry. The new minister in her enthusiasm had changed the allocation of work between the two additional secretaries, me and Shailaja Chandra, without consulting the secretary P.P. Chauhan. He and the MoS had a tough exchange of views before the original work allocation was restored. Chauhan made it clear to me that my major area of work was in NACO though I had to oversee other national disease control programmes such as tuberculosis (TB), leprosy and blindness control. He assured me that as PD NACO I had all the delegated powers of a secretary and would have a free hand in running the programme. He just wanted to be periodically kept informed of any new initiative taken by me. For some reason he did not give me the Malaria programme which remained with the other Additional Secretary, Shailaja Chandra. I was relieved that I did not become a target of a Minister and Secretary tussle as the matter got ironed out before my joining the ministry.

But my heart sank when I tried to look for my NACO team after taking charge. I assumed there would be a strong team leading the national effort to control a virulent epidemic like AIDS. But to my dismay I inherited only a handful of them scattered in remote corners of Nirman

Bhavan, the headquarters of Health Ministry. An Additional Director was heading the technical wing supported by just two mid-level functionaries. A Joint Director from the Indian Information Service was heading the Information Education and Communication (IEC) and prevention work with one consultant to support her. The team was supported by a small finance and administration wing run mostly by consultants. The entire technical team provided by WHO's Global Programme on AIDS (GPA) for technical support to NACO was withdrawn after the GPA was wound up and responsibility for controlling the epidemic was passed on to UNAIDS, the Joint UN Programme on AIDS in 1994/95. The Additional Director informed me that NACO was recently shifted from its spacious accommodation in Red Cross Building in Central Delhi to make room for the newly created Department of Indigenous Systems of Medicine, AYUSH headed by an independent secretary.

I made it a priority to meet the first PD NACO, Pronab Dasgupta, who established the organisation in 1992 and gave it an identity. He was heading the Ministry of Education as Secretary when I met him and was quite candid about his assessment of AIDS response. He told very enthusiastically about the initial efforts at control of the epidemic with the launch of the first phase of the national programme (NACP I) but felt that it still remained largely a health sector programme. He wanted the programme to become truly multisectoral to make an impact. After meeting with him and taking a briefing from officials in NACO it did not take me long to realise that I walked into a battle without even the basic weapons. And little did I anticipate at that time that my time and efforts for the next two decades will be dedicated to fighting a virus that had until now eluded a cure and confounded researchers trying to develop a preventive vaccine.

CHAPTER 1

INITIAL YEARS OF AIDS RESPONSE IN INDIA

When the first cases of human immunodeficiency virus (HIV) were reported in 1986, India was well prepared to monitor its spread, thanks to the initiative taken by the Indian Council of Medical Research (ICMR). Some of the earliest reported cases of acquired immunodeficiency syndrome (AIDS) among Indians were reported in May 1986; one had received blood transfusion and the other received blood product infusion; both cases had been infected out of India. Another seropositive case was detected in a commercial sex worker in Chennai in southern India. These reports sounded the warning bells that HIV had entered India. In May 1986, ICMR AIDS Task Force recommended that a national sero-surveillance programme for screening high-risk and vulnerable groups for HIV infection should be initiated. It was decided that the national surveillance would be established as a collaborative effort of ICMR, Directorate General of Health Services (DGHS), and State Health Authorities. In 6 months, ICMR established a network of 5 reference centres and 43 surveillance centres. By that time it was clear that in India,

1. HIV infection was occurring through all known modes of transmission.
2. HIV infection was present in all the recognised high-risk groups and general population in all states of the country, both in urban and rural areas.
3. Prevalence of HIV infection was relatively high in the high-risk groups; highest prevalence was reported in injecting drug users; female sex workers had the second highest prevalence.
4. Prevalence of HIV infection in general population was still very low.

In India specific guidelines were drawn up and widely disseminated for all priority areas of intervention, most prominently, for care of HIV-infected persons and AIDS patients; pre- and post-test counselling and follow-up care for persons seeking voluntary testing; antenatal, natal, and post-natal care for seropositive mothers; contraceptive care for seropositive women; infants and young children breast-fed by seropositive mothers; immunisation of infants born to seropositive mothers; and infection control and waste management to prevent accidental infection during health care.

However, the efforts of government were mostly confined to monitoring the spread of the epidemic and creating general awareness among people. The efforts were patchy and did not touch even the fringe of the problem. Leaders and people in charge of Ministry of Health were talking in international fora that AIDS will not affect India because of its high moral values! The Global Programme on AIDS (GPA) warned that India had a huge problem on hand and could potentially end up with a high disease burden if proper prevention efforts were not taken. The civil society was raising the alarm bells with high level of mortality setting in urban pockets such as Mumbai and Chennai. It took nearly 6 years for the government to realise the seriousness of the problem.

In 1992, the Ministry of Health asked for the services of Pronab Ranjan (PR) Dasgupta, a senior Indian Administrative Service (IAS) officer who at that time was serving on a World Bank assignment with the Government of Uganda as Health Management Advisor. He got relieved from his assignment to join as the Additional Secretary to look after the AIDS programme in July 1992. Dasgupta was already aware of the HIV outbreak in India while he was serving as Joint Secretary in the Ministry of Health and Family Welfare in 1986. When Prime Minister Rajiv Gandhi was alerted by the DG ICMR Prof. Ramalingaswamy about the seropositive report of the Chennai sex worker, Dasgupta was given the task of preparing a brief for a meeting with the PM.

When he rejoined the Ministry in 1992, the Health Secretary Rajiv Mishra gave him the mandate of choosing a good management model to administer the national programme. After studying various mechanisms existing in the government at that time, Dasgupta favoured the autonomous model of the Space and Atomic Energy Commissions which enjoyed delegated powers of the Ministry of Finance in managing the finances of the programmes. In February 1992, the National AIDS Control Organisation (NACO) was established as a wing of the Ministry of Health with administrative and financial autonomy which became a unique management model to administer a national health programme. The three-tier governance structure established under the model consisted of a National AIDS Committee for policy setting and overseeing the programme at the apex level headed by the Minister of Health and Family Welfare and included both government and nongovernment members. A national AIDS management board headed by the health secretary functioned as the executive board for NACO with all powers of the Ministry of Finance for releasing funds and creating staff positions in the organisation. The third tier was the NACO to be headed by a senior civil servant of the rank of an Additional Secretary as the Project Director. The position enjoyed all delegated powers of a secretary to Government of India. Since then NACO was headed by 16 project directors and the position was re-designated as Director General in 2005. The management structure established in 1992 withstood the test of time and remained relevant even now as the best example of managing a national effort for disease control in India.

FIRST PHASE OF NATIONAL RESPONSE: 1992 TO 1997

The first phase of the National AIDS Control Programme (NACP) got a head start in 1992 under the new management and leadership of Dasgupta. The project was mainly focused on prevention of HIV epidemic with the involvement of all states and union territories by promoting interventions among risk groups, controlling spread of sexually transmitted infections (STIs), cleaning the blood transfusion services and developing capacity to regularly monitor the epidemic. The project adopted a multipronged strategy with five components which were mainly aimed at achieving these objectives.

For the first time, the World Bank came forward to finance a major part of the programme, making it the largest investment by the bank in India's health sector at that time. The World Health Organization (WHO) joined the effort by providing technical support. The project was estimated to cost $99.6 million at the time of appraisal; financed by a government contribution of $14.1 million (Rs. 359.6 million), an International Development Association (IDA) credit of 84.0 million, and a WHO co-financing grant of $1.5 million. The project was originally designed for the 5-year period from 1992 to 1997, but due to slow implementation at start-up, it was extended by 18 months in order to enhance programme's capacity building and institutional strengthening to promote sustainability. With the extension it was able to meet most targets and the credit was closed on March 31, 1999.

The WHO support to the programme through the Global Programme on AIDS (GPA) was a crucial factor in strengthening the technical content of the response in the first phase of the project. NACO was supported by a qualified technical team consisting foreign and Indian technical staff who developed guidelines and protocols for various interventions ranging from testing, blood screening, confidentiality, serosurveillance and sentinel surveillance. A total of 45,000 public sector physicians and 7500 private sector physicians were trained from all over the country in managing AIDS cases and treating opportunistic infections. They were called physicians responsible for AIDS management (PRAM) and were the founding pillars for providing treatment care and support to the large infected population in India. Serosurveillance was carried out with the help of 140 centres located in various hospitals across the country which helped in determining the nature of AIDS epidemic in India and provided invaluable data on the mode of transmission and the hotspots where prevalence of HIV was high. The surveillance data has shown that India's HIV epidemic was driven mainly through the heterosexual route except in North East where injecting drug use was the main risk factor. The states that were impacted most by the heterosexual epidemic were Tamil Nadu and Maharashtra, and by injecting-drug use were Manipur and Nagaland. The early results of surveillance had enabled NACO to focus its efforts on these states.

The project achieved certain specific objectives namely capacity building in AIDS treatment, control of STIs and promotion of use of safe blood. But it was difficult to assess the project's contribution in decelerating the spread of HIV. In 1998, the cumulative infection rate for all HIV tests had shown an increase up to 2.3% from 1% in 1992. But the rates showed a rapid rise in all groups whose behaviours placed them at high risk as HIV continued to spread rapidly in all states of India, constituting a grave development challenge for the country.

I consider the cleaning up of blood safety system in the country as a major achievement of NACP I. As unsafe blood transfusions also accounted for a significantly high proportion of infections, government transferred the responsibility for blood safety to NACO taking it out of the control of DGHS in 1994. State and Union Territories played a major role in providing basic infrastructure facilities, monitoring and coordination of blood bank management. Public sector and voluntary blood banks, of which 815 were strengthened and 154 zonal blood-testing centres established to provide linkages with other blood banks had exceeded the original target. Mandatory HIV screening for all blood transfusions and testing of all blood units for HIV and hepatitis B were introduced, in addition to testing for malaria and syphilis. As a result, blood safety measures increased from 30% in 1992 to virtual universal coverage by the end of the project, exceeding the original target of 90%. Professional/paid donations were totally prohibited by law exceeding the original target calling for a reduction of 30%.

Unexpected support came from India's Supreme Court which delivered a detailed judgement in a Public Interest Litigation (PIL)–Common Cause versus Union of India (1992), on cleaning up blood transfusion system in the country. This judgement helped in phasing out unlicensed blood banks by May 1997, and professional blood donors by December 1997, ensuring availability of safe blood through voluntary donations to people at large.

For implementing the court's order, NACO constituted National and State Blood Transfusion Councils and introduced mandatory testing of blood for HIV along with malaria, syphilis and hepatitis B. The Councils which were tripartite bodies consisting of government, civil society and transfusion experts played a crucial role in raising public awareness about the importance of voluntary donations and provision of safe uninfected blood to patients. When I took charge, the Councils had just started their work and a Joint Director in NACO was looking after the blood safety programme. The mandatory testing of blood for HIV in blood banks was started in full swing and the unlinked anonymous testing for HIV achieved high degree of acceptability among the people and policy makers. The percentage of voluntary donations maintained a steady increase. These initial efforts to clean the blood safety system set the tone for important changes brought during the second phase of NACP.

But NACP I did not measure up to expectations on establishing linkages with civil society and key affected communities. Prevention interventions were very few and not implemented to scale. Condom promotion and M&E systems were also weak at the state level. The reason for this was the constitution of State AIDS Cells with staff drawn from different government departments. The staff was more comfortable working on blood safety and STI control rather than on IEC and community participation.

By the time I joined NACO in July 1997, the first phase of project should have been technically completed. But due to slow implementation of the project during later years and suboptimal fund release and utilisation, the project was extended up to March 1999, lagging by 18 months behind the original completion date. I was literally running the last 18 months of NACP I without any assurance of its continuance. The programme was facing an uncertain future as critics started finding fault with the outcomes and with NACO for not being able to stem the tide of the epidemic. Despite impressive achievements on various components of the programme, the epidemic had shown no signs of abating. What was earlier confined to a few states in southern and North East India had now assumed epidemic proportions in the entire country. Later estimates showed that India was going through the peak of the epidemic in 1997 and 1998. Various estimates were floating around about the number of infections in the absence of a credible estimation process. The sentinel surveillance system introduced in the first phase was not effectively implemented due to lack of involvement and motivation in many states. Frequent transfers of officials at the state and central level affected continuity of the response.

The World Bank which was the main funding agency of NACP I had not expressed clearly whether they would support a second phase. Whomever I spoke with, whether in the government or civil society, were expressing doubts if NACO would continue to implement the response or would be amalgamated with the DGHS. Bringing it back into Nirman Bhavan was also thought as the preliminary step in that direction. I started getting this strange feeling that I was brought there to preside over the liquidation of an organisation midway into achieving control of one of the deadliest epidemics!

Two important events happened in quick succession which strengthened my resolve to stay on and fight for the cause. Within a couple of weeks after my joining, I was asked to lead 14-member delegation to visit Thailand and study the AIDS response there. Thailand was already in the news for the success it achieved in stemming the tide of a raging HIV epidemic fueled mainly by unprotected sex through the sex workers and their clients in Bangkok, Chiang Mai and other urban areas. The trip was sponsored by UNAIDS and a young doctor from Chennai, Sundar Sundararaman, was put as coordinator for the visit. Sundar was running a civil society organisation, AIDS Research Foundation of India (ARFI), in Chennai and was one of the earliest physicians treating AIDS cases in Chennai.

The group was totally unknown to me but everyone was keen to learn from the Thailand experience. Our trip lasted for 5 days. We met senior government officials and community members from the sex worker organisations who were operating from Patpong, one of the large sex worker communities in Bangkok. Our most impactful visit was to the office of Mechai Viravaidya, who as Health Minister of Thailand demystified condoms, the main prevention tools available for preventing the HIV epidemic. Mechai was known as the 'condom man' and his 100% condom promotion campaign was largely responsible for Thailand's success in controlling the heterosexual epidemic. A visit to the restaurant 'Cabbages and Condoms' run by his organisation was enough to understand his foresight in getting the message across that condoms were not forbidden items meant for sexual pleasure but essential tools to protect from HIV and other STIs.

On the third day of our visit, we were taken to Chiang Mai. We met several HIV-positive persons who spoke to us about their work at drop-in centres and through telephonic counselling. Most of our team members met such a large group of openly living HIV-positive persons for the first time. It was a new experience. What impressed me was the cool and matter-of-fact way they talked to us about their health condition and how they were coping with that.

On the last day of our stay, we visited a hospice run by a Buddhist monk for terminally ill AIDS patients. He was taking care of them by treating their opportunistic infections. We later visited an orphanage for children infected by HIV. We saw a room where trained nurses were taking care of about 20 HIV-positive children, all less than 5 years of age. We were asked to get into the room and meet them. Only three members of our team ventured to step in. As I entered, one of the nurses came and offered me to hold a child. I was completely taken by surprise and in reflex action took the child into my arms. That was the first time I had touched an HIV-infected person. The child was a 1-year-old Thai girl! The nurse told that most of these children would not survive for more than 5 years. Except for opportunistic infections, no other treatment was available for HIV-infected children at that time. 'Is this child destined to die'? The cold reality shook me and I could not recover from the shock for most of the day. This encounter moved me deeply and strengthened my resolve to stay and fight instead of getting intimidated by the enormity of the problem.

The Thailand visit had an impact of varying degrees on most of the members and provided us an opportunity to think afresh on our priorities in India. The focused prevention programmes of Thai government implemented with participation of sex worker communities were very impressive. The quiet assurance of HIV-positive persons who organised themselves into communities and the confidence they built up for empowering themselves were worth emulating. It also taught us that we cannot afford a runaway epidemic in India which, given the size of our population, would cost millions of lives of adults and children.

The second incident was a visit to Mumbai I undertook in October 1997, along with Health Secretary Chauhan. The city was already getting branded as the AIDS capital of India with large number of infections reported among sex workers and their clients. We travelled to Mumbai and went on a visit to Kamatipura, the sex worker area commonly known in India as 'red light district'. That was my first visit to a sex worker locality which was quite huge. Estimations varied about the number of sex workers living there which could be anywhere between 80,000 and 100,000. We saw them in unbearable living conditions without even basic civic facilities. For Brihanmumbai Municipal Corporation (BMC) this area was like a dark spot that virtually did not exist on their map. The inhabitants were not provided even a ration card or an electoral registration card which were the basic rights of every Indian. The living conditions were abominable. The place had small rooms, resembling a railway compartment with two or three tiers of beds where they entertained clients with only a piece of cloth separating them from each other. We went there with some of the peer educators from their community. They were very shy to come and speak to us. They were covering their faces when someone tried to take pictures. This was where they entertained four to five clients each in a day on an average. Hundreds of thousands of men–migrant workers from other states of India, those returning from gulf countries and many others with disposable incomes and a craving for paid sex constituted the clientale of this sex worker colony.

Later, in the offices of the BMC we were introduced to a small intervention programme called 'Asha Project'. It was run by the BMC and covered about 5000 sex workers. It was funded by Swedish International Development Agency (SIDA). Compared to the size of Kamatipura population, it was a drop in the ocean, but a brave attempt by the BMC to make a dent in controlling the epidemic in the city. That was where I got the first data on prevalence level of HIV among Mumbai sex workers. But it did not come from any epidemiologist but from one of the peer educators of Asha project. When asked how many people might have already been infected, she replied, 'Saab, samjho aath anna to gaya' (sir, you can assume that 50% are already infected). I thought she was trying to overstate the case. A year later the first national level sentinel data showed that the prevalence of HIV in sex workers in Mumbai was indeed 55%!

The Director of Health Services of the state of Maharashtra, Subhash Salunke, was present in the meeting and informed us of another serious issue, the blockage of sanctioned funds from NACO at the state-government level. Under NACP I, each state had an AIDS cell headed by a technical functionary from the State Directorate of Health Services. Project funds from NACO for implementation of programmes were first released to the state finance departments who in turn released them to the implementors (state AIDS cells) in the health departments. As states of India always had a ways-and-means problem of not carrying adequate funds in their treasury to meet routine government expenditure, they regularly used to divert programme funds received under centrally sponsored projects to meet exigencies, and in the process delay release of funds for priority programmes. The time lag between release by NACO and to the state implementing agencies was anywhere between 3 and 6 months, which resulted in slowing down of implementation.

The visit, the horrific living conditions of Kamatipura's sex workers and most importantly–the level of infections and the inadequacy of response, all weighed down heavily on me. The health secretary also appeared to be pretty shaken by the reality. Both of us did not talk during the entire flight while returning to Delhi. I was trying to gauge the extent of the problem. If 50% of the 100,000 sex workers who are HIV-positive entertain four to five clients every day, how many people must be getting infected daily? The numbers were mind boggling and I stopped calculating.

Back in Delhi, I got the firm conviction that I needed accurate data on the extent of the epidemic and its impact. The sero surveillance done under NACP I could only throw light on the mode of transmission among reported cases which were about 90,000 and the government was reporting this number to the parliament and media. No credible estimates were available on the total number of infections, that is, the prevalence of the epidemic in the country.

The UNAIDS was, however, using a figure of 4.5 to 5 million estimated infections, but these numbers were based on inadequate data from the field. The government was not accepting it as a credible figure. Unless the government comes out with a credible alternative estimate, the UNAIDS figure would get accepted by default. India was already getting branded as the next AIDS capital based on these estimations which were not owned by the government nor were they arrived at with government's participation.

My first task was to get the numbers right. Mohammed Shaukat, the Central Health Service (CHS) officer, in charge of strategic information in NACO briefed me on the problem. The sentinel surveillance system which was put in position under NACP Phase 1 failed to take off due to indifferent participation by majority of the states. The system required collection of blood samples from high-risk groups and general population at regular intervals uniformly across the country. The samples had to be collected by using the unlinked and anonymous method where the identity of the person was kept confidential and no tracing back could be done if that person was found HIV-positive. But the states were doing the survey at their own pace and were not following the protocols developed by NACO. While high-prevalence states such as Maharashtra and Tamil Nadu were systematic in conducting the surveys, others were erratic and irregular. The total number of sites for collection of data was only 54, totally inadequate for the size of the country. Besides NACO was not getting national data collected during the same time slot in all the states in order to make a fair estimate of HIV prevalence in India.

For the next few months, I focused my efforts on getting all the states agree on a common time frame for collection and analysis of data for sentinel surveillance. The number of sites for high-risk groups and general population was also increased to 176.

I constituted a national level steering committee with technical experts to ensure uniformity and quality control in conducting the national level survey. Dr. L.M. Nath, former director of all India Institute of Medical Sciences (AIIMS), was invited to chair the committee. The first national level surveillance was completed in April 1998; 12 years after the first AIDS case was reported in the country!

The results of the survey (Table 1) gave us a clear picture of the extent of spread of the epidemic in the country and since then formed the basis for an evidence-based national AIDS response. The surveys were repeated every year and the number of sites was progressively increased to 384 by 2002 and 1359 by 2010.

■ Table 1: Results of first sentinel surveillance survey (August to October 1998)

Sl. No.	States	No. of Sites	HIV Prevalence in Percent	
			Range	Median
1	Andhra Pradesh	ANC-4	1.50 to 2.75	2.25
		STD-4	9.60 to 34.80	23.10
2	Andaman and Nicobar	ANC-1	0	0
		STD-1	0	0
3	Arunachal Pradesh	ANC-1	0 to 0.40	0.40
		STD-2	0	0
4	Assam	ANC-2	0	0
		STD-2	0.40 to 3.08	1.74
5	Bihar	ANC-3	0	0
		STD-4	0.39 to 1.65	1.35
6	Chandigarh	ANC-1	0 to 2.50	0.47
		STD-2	0 to 5.91	2.95
7	Dadra and Nagar Haveli	ANC-1	0	0
8	Daman and Diu	ANC-2	0 to 0.26	0.13
		STD-1	0	0
9	Delhi	ANC-2	0.25	0.25
		STD-1	1.60	1.60
10	Goa	ANC-2	0.73 to 1.73	1.23
		STD-2	16 to 23.01	19.50
11	Gujarat	ANC-2	0	0
		STD-2	1.78 to 3.30	2.54
12	Haryana	ANC-1	0	0
		STD-1	2.60	2.60
13	Himachal Pradesh	ANC-2	0.24 to 0.49	0.36
		STD-3	0 to 0.40	0.39
14	Jammu and Kashmir	STD-1	0	0
		ANC-2		
15	Karnataka	ANC-1	1.75	1.75
		STD-7	5.95 to 40.32	16.41
16	Kerala	ANC-3	0 to 0.20	0.10
		STD-5	0 to 4.51	2.60
17	Lakshadweep	STD-1	0 to 1.30	0.65
		ANC-2		
18	Madhya Pradesh	ANC-6	0 to 0.94	0.47
		STD-4	0 to 4.35	2.59
19	Maharashtra	ANC-12	0 to 5	2.37
		STD-8	4.80 to 50.80	16
20	Manipur	ANC-5	0.75 to 3.50	0.75
		STD-2	6.20 to 6.30	4.15
		IDU-3	70.33 to 76.09	70.73

Sl. No.	States	No. of Sites	HIV Prevalence in Percent	
			Range	Median
21	Meghalaya	ANC-2	0 to 0.25	0.13
		STD-2	0	0
22	Mizoram	ANC-2	0 to 0.96	0.48
		STD-1	1.49	1.19
		IDU-1	1	1
23	Nagaland	ANC-4	0.50 to 1.25	0.70
		STD-1	11.10	11.10
		IDU-1	13.20	13.20
24	Orissa	ANC-2	0	0
		STD-2	0 to 3	1.50
25	Pondicherry (Puducherry)	STD-1	7.20	7.20
		ANC-1	0.50	0.50
26	Punjab	ANC-2	0	0
		STD-2	1 to 2.60	1.80
27	Rajasthan	ANC-3	0	0
		STD-2	4.40 to 6	5.22
28	Sikkim	ANC-2	0 to 0.25	0.13
		STD-1	0	0
29	Tamil Nadu	ANC-5	0.50 to 3	1
		STD-3	8 to 23	16
30	Tripura	ANC-1	0	0
		STD-1	0	0
31	Uttar Pradesh	ANC-6	0 to 0.25	0.24
		STD-4	1.20 to 3.30	1.60
32	West Bengal	ANC-4	0.25 to 0.75	0.62
		STD-4	0.80 to 2.39	2

Abbreviations: ANC, antenatal care; STD, sexually transmitted disease.
Source: Project Implementation Plan, NACP Phase II, National AIDS Control Organisation.

While Tamil Nadu, Manipur and Maharashtra were known earlier as high prevalence states, the other two southern states, Andhra Pradesh and Karnataka, also reported high prevalence levels both in high-risk groups and general population. This was surprising information. Three different levels of epidemic were noticed from the results of the survey (1) the high prevalence group with Maharashtra and Southern India and Manipur, (2) the medium prevalence with Gujarat, West Bengal and Nagaland and (3) rest of the country as of low prevalence.

After getting the prevalence levels, we set upon the task of estimating the total number of infections prevailing in the country. This is a new task for the epidemiologists. We invited two external experts to advise us on the estimation process, James Chin from the University of Berkeley and Karen Stanecki from the US Bureau of Census.

The team finally came up with an estimated figure of 3 million infections among adults in India. Our worst fears had come true. The country was witnessing a raging HIV epidemic second only to South Africa, but only about 90,000 cases were getting reported! The challenging task was to explain the huge difference between the reported and estimated cases to the policy makers. More difficult was the task to announce the numbers to the people, the parliament and the media who until then were only provided the reported figures of less than a 100,000.

The Minister of State for Health who was from a regional party in Tamil Nadu had taken the plunge and made an official announcement that India had a serious HIV epidemic and about 3 million people were already infected making it the country with the second highest prevalence after South Africa. Given the extreme level of denial that was existing in the country on AIDS, we thought it was not enough to get an announcement from the Ministry of Health. The message had to come from the highest political functionary, the Prime Minister (PM) of India. We sought an audience with the PM Atal Bihari Vajpayee, to brief him and request him to make a policy announcement on AIDS with the latest prevalence figures. Atal ji was the greatest leader of his time and could grasp the seriousness of the issue in 15 minutes of discussion. In his characteristic style he gave a long pause and said, '*sach ko logon ke samne jaroor le aana chahiye*'. (It is important to make people aware of this truth.) In December 1998, the strongest endorsement came from PM Vajpayee who called it 'India's most important public health problem' in a meeting of the parliamentarians. India finally came out of the denial mode.

I view this announcement as a landmark and a game changer in India's AIDS control efforts. For the next 10 to 12 years the country never looked back in its determined response to bring the epidemic under control and finally succeeded in reversing the increasing trend. But the day after the announcement, all hell broke loose in the media with many newspapers reporting it as front-page news. There was bitter criticism from both extremes, some blaming the government for living in denial so long and another section seeing a conspiracy to bring 'foreign' money into India for what they called an 'exaggerated public health problem'. For the next few days NACO had a tough time answering these critics which took our time and energy. I was in one way happy that for once AIDS was recognised as a public health priority by the media and started engaging national attention. For the next 10 years it stayed as a high public health priority and attracted political and financial support for its response.

The announcement also produced great relief among the global players who were grappling with the problem of convincing the government that India had a higher prevalence of HIV than what was getting reported. Executive Director UNAIDS and the World Bank lead manager congratulated the government for biting the bullet and accepting the seriousness of the problem.

Our next challenge was to get global support for the national HIV estimation process. The Asia Pacific Conference on AIDS in Asia Pacific (ICAAP) held in Kuala Lumpur in 1999 provided us an opportunity to exchange India's national surveillance data and HIV estimation methodology with the Monitoring of AIDS Pandemic (MAP) group in UNAIDS. Peter Piot, invited us to present the national estimations before the group headed by Bernhard Schwartländer the head of the epidemiology division in UNAIDS. The estimation process and the robustness of the national estimates received endorsement from the group as it was based on credible primary data emerging out of the first national sentinel surveillance conducted in 1998. The estimation process undertaken by NACO was an inclusive and transparent one as it involved technical personnel from UNAIDS, WHO and the World Bank along with national experts. Since then India's national estimates were always jointly prepared and announced by NACO and UNAIDS and got incorporated in the global estimates published every year by UNAIDS.

CHAPTER 2

NATIONAL AIDS CONTROL PROGRAMME, PHASE II

The extended period of the National AIDS Control Programme (NACP) phase 1 was getting over and there was overall apprehension about continuation of national AIDS programme. My next task was to set at rest all speculations and ensure that funding support would continue for the national programme both from domestic and external sources.

The bold step Government of India (GOI) had taken in owning the large number of 3 million infections had also encouraged the donors to renew their commitment to finance a second phase of NACP. The World Bank team comprising Richard Skolnik, Salim Habayeb and Prabhat Jha had started the concept review for NACP II in January 1999, and major donors viz Department for International Development (DFID) of United Kingdom, U.S. Agency for International Development (USAID) and Canadian International Development Agency (CIDA) joined the project. The Joint United Nations Programme on HIV/AIDS (UNAIDS) had assured technical support for project preparation. In the next few months I had plunged headlong into a hectic schedule of activity in National AIDS Control Organisation (NACO) for preparation of the new project. Visits by UNAIDS and the World Bank officials became frequent and we only had a limited number of persons in NACO to engage them.

PROJECT PREPARATION FOR NACP II

We therefore constituted a project preparation team with Sundararaman, Subhash Salunke, Ramasundaram, who was the Project Director (PD) of Tamil Nadu State AIDS Control Society (TNSACS) and Subhash Hira,

Director of AIDS Research and Control Centre (ARCON), Mumbai, as Technical Liaison Officers (TLOs). The project formulation for NACP II followed a truly participatory approach. Between April and June 1998, the TLOs in collaboration with State AIDS Cells, conducted state-level planning workshops in all the states and in the cities of Mumbai, Chennai and Ahmedabad with involvement of all major stakeholders. This was a stupendous task performed in a record time with involvement of the state governments and civil society partners. I was keeping close contact with the TLOs and other members of the NACO team involved in project preparation. That was one of the most intensive phases of project preparation and the overall energy and enthusiasm of stakeholders was exemplary. Visits by the World Bank officials, UNAIDS technical teams and bilateral donors kept us busy but the high motivation levels of my colleagues kept us at pace with the demands of work.

By end of June 1998, the first drafts of state level project implementation plans (PIPs) started taking shape. This was followed by a series of state-level and national-level workshops to ensure identification of right priorities for the project and filling up of all gaps in implementation strategies. Technical resource groups (TRGs) were established for 12 different thematic areas to provide technical assistance to the states and implementing agencies. They were located in institutions specialised in the area of technical expertise and supported by experts with proven track record.

The responsibilities of various stakeholders in the national effort were clearly delineated in the national PIP (Table 2) which was finally presented to the World Bank and other agencies in January 1999.

For me, getting more funds for the second phase was important but ensuring a smooth flow of funds to the states and the implementing agencies at the field level was equally a critical task. The most important institution for delivery of services, the State AIDS Cells were the weakest link in the entire chain. These were small units located within the State Directorates of Health Services and normally headed by a very junior functionary in the hierarchy in the rank of a joint director. In the state bureaucracy, the functionary needed to go through at least three or four tiers to get to the policy-making level of the minister or the secretary. The availability of funds for programmes was more challenging. Under the existing dispensation NACO released programme funds to the state finance departments who in turn channelised them to the state programme cells. This lengthy process resulted in delays to reach funds to implementing units. The heads of the State AIDS Cells did not have sufficient clout in the government to get the process expedited.

■ **Table 2:** Participation of agencies in NACP II preparation. The responsibilities of the various agencies under the project can be described in the following 'who does what' table[a]:

Name of the Agency	Responsibilities of the Agency
National AIDS Committee	National policy making
National AIDS Control Board	Approval of national annual action plans and formation of project management teams.
National AIDS Control Organization	Policy planning, strategy development, coordination between donors and implementing agencies, procurement, operational research, research and development and monitoring and evaluation
State and MC AIDS Control Societies	Formulation, implementation and monitoring of project activities, ensuring adherence to PFMS, coordination between local implementing agencies like public sector, NGOs, private sector, panchayat institutions etc.
TRGs	Provide technical assistance to the State and MC level and ACSs in the implementation of their activities
Existing Public Sector Medical and Health Institutions	Direct service delivery such as blood banking, STD control serivces, VTCs, clinical care and support of PLWAs, Training, O.R. and R.D.
Nongovernment Agencies	Implementation of the PTIs, community and home-based care and running of hospices for PLWAs, Providing counselling in VTCs.
UNAIDS	Financial and technical support to TRGs
Other UN agencies	Implement AIDS control activities relevant to their sector
Bilaterals	Collaboration with NACO, State and MC ACSs, NGOs, private sector

Abbreviations: MC ACS, Municipal Corportaion AIDS Control societies; NGOs, nongovernmental organisations; O.R., operations research; PFMS; project finance and moitoring suystems; PTI, priority-trgeted interventions; R.D., research and development; STD, sexually transmitted disease; TRGs, technical resource groups; VTCs, voluntary testing centres.
[a] While the above table gives an overview of who does what, the activity-specific process/sub-process tables in Annex-x give a more detailed picture of the level of implementation, implementing agency, person(s) responsible for implantation for every major activity under the project. (Ref: Annex-x)
Source: Project Implementation Phase of National AIDS Control Programme II, page 36.

One exception to this scenario was Tamil Nadu, a southern state with high HIV prevalence. While other states were struggling to get funds for implementation, Tamil Nadu could access and utilise funds quickly and also devise innovative programmes for awareness and HIV prevention. The management model adopted in the state was itself an innovative structure in governance and facilitated smooth release of funds for programme implementation. This experiment had a history behind it.

During NACP I, USAID developed a bilateral AIDS Prevention and Control (APAC) project focusing on the high-risk groups in Tamil Nadu. A tripartite implementation mechanism was developed in consultation with GOI, Government of Tamil Nadu (GOTN) and USAID. Voluntary health services (VHS), a reputed nongovernmental organisation (NGO) in the area of health care was chosen for fund management and utilisation by civil society partners. But the funds released by NACO to state treasury units were not reaching the state AIDS cell. It was then decided to have a direct transfer of bilateral funds to the implementation units of VHS from GOI. But unfortunately, the process took almost 2 years to get the necessary GOI clearances and the APAC project could not take off on schedule. Finally APAC project began functioning in mid-1995. During this period, GOTN was also keen to access the USAID funds and quickly decided to set up an autonomous body to be managed by a committee headed by the health secretary. Thus, GOTN established the Tamil Nadu State AIDS Control Society (TNSACS) with an Indian Administrative Service (IAS) officer as a Project Director (PD). The TNSACS was registered under the Society Registration Act with a three-tier structure of a general body, a management board and a PD as chief executive officer responsible for carrying its operations. It was the first time this model was adopted to manage a major public health programme in India. The leadership provided by successive PDs such as Purnalingam, Ramasundaram, Allauddin and their successors, who were senior IAS officers in the state government, contributed to successful implementation of national AIDS programmes in Tamil Nadu. Tamil Nadu society was also the first to take the initiative to recruit an HIV-positive person as an employee in the society office and to include an HIV-positive person in the governing board of the society.

In our discussion with the World Bank officials we agreed to adopt the Tamil Nadu society model with necessary strengthening and improvement in all states. The NACP II project team was asked to develop a management structure based on the Tamil Nadu society model and estimate the requirement of staff and other infrastructural needs. The project team did a commendable job in formulating the proposal and in less than a year 28 SACS were constituted and registered. Important ones were provided full-time services of senior-level IAS officers from the state governments. This large-scale expansion of the implementation machinery involved creation of more than 700 technical and operational positions in all the societies and in NACO. In a normal government process it would have taken several months to get the financial approvals for such a large number of staff. The management board of NACO had the powers to create positions without the formal approval of the Ministry of Finance under NACO's delegation orders issued in 1992. But these powers were never utilised earlier. I decided to explore this option and got support from the health secretary who headed the board and the finance ministry representative on the board. The National AIDS Control Board (NACB) sanctioned the 700-contractual positions in a single government order for all the 28 state societies and NACO. Now the organisational machinery for implementation of NACP II was in position.

The State AIDS Control Societies (SACS) on an average consisted of a staff strength of 25 to 30 depending upon the size and population of the state. The PD should be a civil servant drawn from IAS and technical staff from state services as joint directors for prevention, care, support and treatment, and IEC. Other key support staff was from operations, finance and M&E. The SACS provided a unique coordination space and opportunity for government, private sector, NGO, PLHA and civil society networks to work together. This innovative model was not tried until then for any public health programme.

The highly participatory process of project preparation also resulted in generating donor interest in the programme. Initially some of the bilateral agencies wanted to directly channel funds to the implementing agencies and were reluctant to pool their resources through the budgetary mechanism of the GOI. This would have created problems of ensuring uniformity in providing services and monitoring the response. We decided to opt for pooling all domestic and external resources through a single budgetary channel to finance NACP II. The World Bank, which was the major financing agency, had also supported this approach. We held separate discussions with major bilateral funders DFID, USAID and CIDA and convinced them about the efficiency gains in a single management structure by pooling funds through the government budgetary system.

Under NACP I, NACO and its partner agencies such as USAID, DFID and AUSAID had implemented a number of intervention programmes, technical support initiatives and pilot projects and identified several best practices in prevention interventions for high-risk groups in condom promotion, STI programs, counselling and behavioural change communications.

The bilateral donors were interested in continuing their work in NACP II also in key focused states where they had a presence for providing technical support to the SACS. This was accomplished through mutual discussion and agreement with the states. DFID was closely working with Kerala and Orissa (Odisha) governments and continued to provide direct technical assistance to their SACS. CIDA expressed preference to support Rajasthan and Karnataka. USAID had agreed to provide funding to Mumbai Society for prevention activities in Mumbai city under AVERT project in addition to the APAC project they were assisting in Tamil Nadu. Australian Agency for International Development (AusAID) with their experience in harm reduction programmes was asked to support the northeastern states. This arrangement had greatly facilitated provision of direct technical assistance to the newly appointed personnel in the SACS with the help of trained experts such as Pradeep Kakkattil, Madhu Deshmukh and Vidhya Ganesh from DFID, Rekha Masilamani and Sudhakar Kurapati from USAID and Nandini Kapoor from AusAID.

With the expanded activity under NACP II, we needed additional workspace for NACO. I started looking for a new building as the space in Nirman Bhavan was inadequate. We found a floor in the New Delhi Municipal Corporation (NDMC) office building in the central Delhi district of Connaught Place and got it refurbished. The 9th floor of Chandralok building became the corporate office of NACO from October 1999. It could provide accommodation to all functionaries in NACO and had common facilities like a conference room. It gave an identity to the organisation and was more accessible to communities and common people who were not required to go through the strict security procedures that were needed for getting into Nirman Bhavan, the headquarters of Ministry of Health. In keeping with the policy of civil society involvement, a separate room was reserved in the building for use by the community representatives. We could get more technical staff and consultants to take up the increased workload in NACO with the project preparation for the second phase of NACP.

NATIONAL AIDS CONTROL POLICY

One serious gap in the national response in India was the absence of a national policy on HIV/AIDS. The World Health Organization (WHO) Global Programme on AIDS (GPA) team did a commendable job in preparing technical guidelines for various components of the national response but a comprehensive national policy on HIV/AIDS was still not in position. Manipur, one of the small states in the north east which was witnessing a severe injecting drug user (IDU)-driven epidemic could develop a state AIDS control policy much earlier in October 1996.

The funding agencies, especially the World Bank, were also expecting a policy paper from the GOI stating the objectives especially on issues such as confidentiality, protection of human rights of persons living with AIDS (PLHAs), and access to prevention and treatment services. I initiated a process of consultations with important stakeholders to draft a national policy which included civil society and community leaders, physicians treating AIDS cases in public and private sector and state government officials implementing the programme. It was a great opportunity to interact with a cross-section of civil society leaders who in one way or the other were involved with HIV/AIDS programmes in India. During the consultation process I interacted closely with pioneers; Anjali Gopalan, Anand Grover, Smarajit Jana, Alka Deshpande, Ishwar Gilada and Suniti Solomon and community leaders such as Ashok Row Kavi, Luke Samson, Neville and Elizabeth Selhore, Ashok Pillai, Ramesh Venkataraman, Mona Mishra and Toghuku Yepthomi to name a few. Their association continued with the programme even at later stages, bringing NACO very close to the community leadership during the implementation phase of NACP II. I could sense an overall anxiety, disillusion and anger among the community leaders for lack of clarity on continuation of the national programme beyond 1997, the end date of NACP I. At times there were heated arguments about provision of care and support and testing facilities for high-risk groups. Every one of those meetings was helpful in identifying the serious gaps in the national response and in putting together a national policy to comprehensively address them.

By the time the project preparation for NACP II neared completion, we could finalise the National AIDS Control Policy and get approval from the minister of health and the National AIDS Committee. The Central Council for Health and Family Welfare (CCHFW), a consultative body of central and state governments on health issues had also endorsed the national policy. That was sufficient for the World Bank and other donors to appreciate the commitment of the government to the second phase of the NACP. In my letter of 7 May 1999 to the Country Director of the World Bank in India, I highlighted the key features of the national policy and confirmed the GOI's support and commitment to implement the policy in all aspects. Even though the policy was still not 'officially' approved by the Union Cabinet, the World Bank recognised the support given by the CCHFW and the Ministry of Health as sufficient to go ahead with appraisal of NACP II and subsequent steps leading to its approval by the Bank Board and GOI in July 1999.

Approval of the Union Cabinet was finally obtained in 2002 to the National AIDS Control Policy and the National Blood Policy, which until today are the guiding policy documents for responding to HIV/AIDS and ensuring safe blood to the people.

Because of the widespread consultation process with all stakeholders and building of consensus it was possible to accommodate all critical aspects of prevention, treatment, testing and multisectoral cooperation in the national policy. It was recognised that prevention of the epidemic among key populations namely sex workers, IDUs, men who have sex with men (MSM) and transgender population was the key to reduction of new infections.

Condoms, safe needles and syringes were advocated as the principal prevention tools. Confidentiality for testing and counselling was given due importance and protection of the rights of HIV-positive people from stigma and discrimination was prominently highlighted. Intersectoral cooperation involving non-health sectors of government and private sector was stressed to address AIDS, not just as a health issue but as an overall development challenge. On the issue of treatment, the civil society groups were agitating for introduction of antiretroviral (ARV) drugs, but the prices of drugs were still prohibitively expensive and the government could not commit antiretroviral therapy (ART) provision in the national policy. There was a promise to review the policy as the prices of ARVs become affordable. Within 1 year after announcing the policy, prices of ARVs came crashing due to the sensational decision of CIPLA and other generic manufacturers in India to make ARVs accessible at a low cost to AIDS patients in India and in the developing world. In December 2003, the GOI kept its promise to review the policy and announced provision of ART to 70,000 AIDS patients to begin with.

JOINT UN PROGRAMME ON AIDS (UNAIDS)

In the run up to formulation of national policy and NACP II, I established close contacts with the Joint Programme of United Nations on AIDS (UNAIDS), which was just 3-years old and had a small secretariat in India. After the GPA of WHO got wound up in 1994, the leadership was passed on to the joint programme with six cosponsoring organisations from the UN system: WHO, United Nations Development Programme (UNDP), UNICEF, International Labour Organization (ILO), United Nations Population Fund (UNFPA) and the World Bank. A Programme Coordinating Board (PCB) functioned as the Board of Management with members drawn from donor and recipient governments and civil society partners selected on a regional basis. It was supported by a secretariat located in Geneva. Dr. Peter Piot, the Belgian microbiologist already famous for his research in Ebola and HIV became its first Executive Director. After helping discover the Ebola virus in 1976 and leading efforts to contain the first-ever recorded Ebola epidemic that same year, Dr. Piot became a pioneering researcher into AIDS and worked in the GPA under the leadership of Jonathan Mann, the renowned

AIDS researcher who was heading the GPA in WHO at that time. He took over the leadership of UNAIDS in 1994 and led the global response to AIDS for the next 14 years.

In October 1997, I first met Peter Piot at the International Conference on AIDS in Asia Pacific (ICAAP) held at Manila. The ICAAPs are biannual events held jointly by regional civil society organisations of Asia Pacific and UNAIDS. Minister of State for Health, Renuka Chowdhary and I as PD NACO represented the government at the conference. For both of us it was the first AIDS conference and provided an opportunity to interact with global and regional players prominent in the AIDS movement. Our first meeting with civil society leaders from India was quite stormy with many of them openly criticising the attitude of the Indian government towards the AIDS challenge. Minister Chowdhary deftly handled the situation and promised an intensified AIDS control programme in the second phase. She introduced me to the participants and expressed confidence in my leadership of NACO. Peter and the conference organisers invited me and Minister Chowdhary to participate in other events in the conference and speak about India's AIDS situation and how the government was handling it.

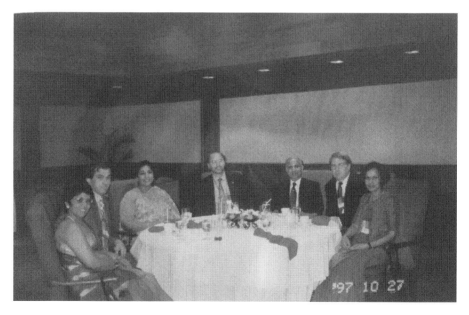

With Minister of State for Health, Renuka Chowdhary (third from left), Peter Piot (fourth from left) and his team at Manila ICAAP 1997

The UNAIDS had a small country office in India with two functionaries and supported by a theme group (TG) of UN cosponsors. The chair of the TG rotated between the cosponsors and the Country Programme Advisor (CPA) from the secretariat functioned under the overall guidance of the TG. The TG chair I first met was Wasim Zaman from UNFPA, a Bangladeshi professional who welcomed me to his office. I was still not clear on the relationship between the TG and the national programme. Wasim Zaman was trying to impress upon me that the TG regularly monitors the national programme in India and would like to get regular inputs from PD NACO. I responded that it was the primary responsibility of the government to address the challenge of the AIDS epidemic in India and the Joint UN programme under the guidance of TG was meant to provide advocacy and technical support to the national programme. He was initially taken aback at this new role definition, but understood the message I was trying to convey. The prime mover of national response had to be the national programme which was accountable to the people and the parliament. Other stakeholders including the joint UN programme need to get meaningfully involved to support the national effort based on their mandates and technical capacities. This was a policy I tried to follow later also as the director of the UNAIDS regional team in Bangkok.

I again met Peter twice in 1998, once in the PCB meetings and second time at the International AIDS Conference held at Geneva. We developed instant rapport and kept in touch regularly. I was impressed by his passion and commitment, but also realised that he had an unenviable task on hand. The debates in the PCB were heated and acrimonious at times with the civil society partners not happy with the treatment programmes which were just unfolding in the North but still very unaffordable in the developing countries of Africa and Asia. Peter was happy to see India's commitment to prevent and control the epidemic and assured full support from UNAIDS. He asked Jim Sherry, his Director of Programme Development, to keep direct liaison with me to provide technical support for NACP II. He brought in Gordon Alexander, Deputy Director in UNICEF India office, as the CPA of UNAIDS to assist the national efforts. Gordon remained a close ally all through the project preparation stage and later during the implementation of NACP II.

PROJECT APPROVAL AND FOLLOW-UP

As the project preparation activities picked up momentum, the World Bank team projected two different sets of approaches for financing the national programme. A section of the bank's staff wanted that the bank should only concern itself with prevention programmes that contribute to bringing down the new infections in the country. This group was averse to continue funding general prevention programmes such as blood safety and treatment of opportunistic infections. It became clear to me that ART programmes were a no go with the bank at that time, due to the prohibitive cost of interventions. I was not convinced with the argument for part funding of certain components of the national programme. As the World Bank's assistance was a soft loan from its International Development Association's (IDA) arm and not an outright grant, it should be made available to the government as budgetary support for the entire programme. We needed to bolster the blood safety network in the country as infected blood accounted for 8% of all infections at that time. Care and support to people living with HIV had to be an important component of the national programme. In one of the discussions with Prabhat Jha, the lead of the World Bank group, I took a firm stand that the assistance from the bank should be for the entire national programme and not be restricted to specific components. After much discussion the bank leadership was convinced of the need to provide across the board funding for all the components of the national programme irrespective of the geographical location and thematic areas of intervention. This was a major step forward and became the guiding principle for all subsequent bank-financed projects in India.

The principled stand we took both with the bank leadership and the joint UN programme drove home the message that the government of India was firmly committed to be in the forefront of AIDS response and be accountable to the people for the success or failure of the national efforts. Financial and technical support from development partners and multilateral agencies should conform to overall government policies and strategies. Experience had shown that whenever national programmes assumed leadership and acted as rallying points for AIDS response, the outcomes were always positive.

With the combined efforts of the project teams of NACO and the World Bank-led external donors, the PIP for NACP II was finally approved by the Expenditure Finance Committee of the GOI in April 1999. I travelled to Washington for negotiations for the IDA credit of $190 million and presented the plan to the World Bank team. Events quickly followed and the credit was approved in June 1999.

Bilateral donors viz DFID, USAID, CIDA and AusAID joined the programme and agreed to route their funding through the government budgetary process making it a truly multisectoral one.

Financial contributions from major stakeholders are given in Table 3.

■ Table 3 Resources budget of NACP II	
Agency	**Contribution (million US $)**
Central government	$92.6
State governments	$221.0
World Bank	$191.1
Bilaterals	$81.2
UNAIDS	$14.4
Others	$10.2
Total	$610.5

The total financial commitment for NACP II was $610.5 million, making it the largest health sector project launched in India for control of a communicable disease at that time. The programme was launched on 31 July 1999, and the IDA credit took effect from November 1999.

I was quite happy with the final outcome secured after 1 year of intensive preparation phase followed by negotiations with the World Bank and other donors and establishment of institutional structures such as the national policy, the SACS, the TRGs and the NGO Advisor network. There was a new wave of enthusiasm in NACO and state governments with many of the state health secretaries enthusiastically participating and lending support to NACO.

The NACP II addressed the principal components of prevention, care and support, multisectoral cooperation and strengthening institutional capacity. The unique feature was the large allocation for priority-targeted interventions for 'groups at high risk'. (The terminology for defining these groups kept changing regularly from high-risk groups to the current term of key populations.) Of the total budget, 23% was allocated for this important component of the programme. The core work was to expand the prevention programme, especially for the high-risk populations, most importantly the sex workers. The impression from my Mumbai visit was still fresh in my memory. We needed to control the heterosexual epidemic which accounted for almost 85% of infections to bring in better control over HIV incidence. The targeted intervention (TI) model had to be standardised in order to launch it and scale up throughout the country. In an intensive workshop held with participation of communities and experts we developed costing models for TIs not just for the risk groups but sections of vulnerable groups namely migrants, transport workers and street children. Swarup Sarkar and Mahesh Mahalingam from UNAIDS provided technical advice and facilitated the costing process. At the end of the workshop we prepared unit costs for all TIs which were to be used as the basis for starting new interventions by the SACS. We also decided to hand over the existing TIs which were directly managed by NACO to the respective state societies. Some of the implementing NGOs were reluctant and apprehensive about doing work with state-level officials, fearing delay and corruption in financial deals. I had to reason it out with them that civil society partners should learn to work with the state societies as NACP II would be a decentralised programme and the states would be in the forefront of AIDS response. They were assured that a large training programme for the SACS officials would be taken up and the band of NGO advisors recruited in the SACS would act as a bridge between the NGO implementors and SACS officials. Officials in SACS, NGOs and civil society organisations (CSOs) were provided detailed training for starting new TIs, including financial management and audit. The NGO advisors who were recruited directly by the SACS with civil society background had played a crucial role not just in sensitising the SACS officials but in monitoring the flow of fund to the implementing agencies. Within a period of 1 year the number of TIs was scaled-up to 700 and by the end of NACP II to 1033.

Prevention among general population, which included blood safety and Information Education and Communication (IEC) campaigns got another large chunk of 33.7% of the programme budget. The total funds spent on prevention thus accounted for 56.7%, one of the highest allocations made for prevention under any national programme. Strengthening institutional capacity received 24.8% and intersectoral collaboration 10.1%. Low-cost AIDS care got 14.1% which included treatment of opportunistic infections and palliative care. The World Bank and other donors were still not ready to finance the ARV treatment programmes as the cost of ARVs was still prohibitively expensive. This remained a sore point in our relations with civil society partners until December 2003 when the first ART programme was launched by NACO.

The overall objective of NACP was to reduce the spread of HIV in India and to strengthen India's capacity to respond to HIV/AIDS in the long-term. When the project came to an end in 2006, both these objectives were achieved in good measure. While India's overall infection rates were not only controlled, but had kept an impressive pace of decline for the next 10 years. The country could strengthen its capacity at various levels, national, state, district and community to sustain the response for the next 20 years. The NACO and its institutional structure remained the strongest disease-control infrastructure for any public health programme in India. The NACP II in many ways laid a solid foundation for a long and sustained response to HIV/AIDS in India.

But it was not a smooth sailing for the programme. It met with an unexpected hurdle even before it was formally launched. A group of women activists led by the wife of a senior constitutional authority wrote to Prime Minister Vajpayee, objecting to the active sex workers' interventions under NACP II. They were alleging that a deeper 'conspiracy' was taking place to legalise sex work in India by empowering the sex workers through the TIs. Prime Minister's Office (PMO) called for a report, but did not ask us to put the project on hold. I was worried whether after all the efforts of the past 2 years, the project might get blocked or shelved altogether. The civil society was angered at this sudden turn of events and demanded a separate meeting to air their grievances before the PM. Their representation was also sent to PMO. Later, neither did we hear anything from PMO about the objections raised by the earlier group nor did we get any direction to put the programme on hold. The programme had other detractors also. The Joint Action Committee, an umbrella grouping of NGOs working in the areas of human rights and HIV, was also campaigning against the NACP II as it targeted so-called high-risk groups, allegedly leading to their social ostracisation. They were seeing a 'deep conspiracy' to justify the expending of all too readily available loans from the World Bank! But the programme continued to receive high-level political support and had a smooth sailing after that.

IMPLEMENTATION PHASE–NACP II

Implementation of NACP II was taken up in right earnest after the launch of the programme. The next 3 years were one of the most intensive periods of field work in my career. The programme had to be implemented from 28 state societies, 10 central ministries and departments and scores of CSOs. External partners ranged from the World Bank and bilateral donors agencies to UNAIDS and its cosponsor organisations in India. The most important supporters for our work were the PMO, parliamentary and legislative assemblies at the central and state level and local bodies such as municipal corporations, panchayat raj agencies at the village, sub-district and district level.

Strengthening the management capacity of NACO and SACS and providing technical support was foremost in my mind for a long and sustained battle against the epidemic. We could attract committed and technically sound professionals into NACO. Neelam Kapur, the Indian Information Service official heading the IEC and TI divisions, took the initiative to recruit committed personnel with civil society background as NGO advisors in SACS who functioned as vital links with CSO and PLHA networks. A new Additional Director, P. L. Joshi, was brought in to supervise the technical work of NACO. Salil Panakadan who worked during NACP I rejoined NACO as Joint Director and assumed charge of the blood safety and monitoring and evaluation work. Mohammed Shaukat continued with strategic information work and developed effective liaison with Geneva-based experts in UNAIDS for conducting periodic sentinel surveillance and preparing national-level estimates for HIV. With 10 new TRGs coming into existence we utilised the technical capacity of the institutions where they were based for strategic support to SACS. A total number of 786,000 persons were provided training in the 5-year period (2000-2005) in various fields of specialisation ranging from physicians, nurses and other health care providers to rural medical practitioners and private doctors.

At the apex level, the National AIDS Committee (NAC) was reconstituted with the health minister as the chair and with representations from state governments, central ministries, civil society partners and medical experts as members. The NAC met regularly and took several strategic initiatives to intensify the response. The National AIDS Control Board (NACB) provided administrative support to NACO. We were fortunate to get excellent guidance and political support from the PMO throughout the implementation phase of the programme. From the time he made the first announcement on HIV prevalence in India, PM Vajpayee was always accessible and provided leadership whenever needed. Midway during the implementation phase we felt that the programme needed a strong political push in the northeastern states. PM Vajpayee gave us time to hold a meeting with the seven chief ministers (CMs) of the states exclusively to discuss performance on the AIDS issue. Since then the CMs started monitoring the programme and were regularly giving feedback to PMO on the progress of implementation. In May 2001, the PM addressed the CMs of the high prevalence states of Maharashtra, Andhra Pradesh, Karnataka, Tamil Nadu, Manipur and Nagaland and exhorted them to give priority to AIDS programmes. On 26 July 2003, he spoke at the national convention of elected representatives and cautioned against complacency. He exhorted the people's representatives to become aware of AIDS problem first and then spread the message of awareness among the people. He reminded them of the wiseman's message 'The best time to plant a tree was 20 years ago. The next best time is now'. PM Vajpayee's leadership during that 5-year period proved very critical for the national AIDS response due to the low political profile of successive health ministers who rotated fast until Health Minister Sushma Swaraj took charge in 2003.

BEHAVIORAL SURVEILLANCE SURVEYS

While the sentinel survey had given us baseline data on the prevalence levels and the total number of infections in the country, the risk factors contributing to the rapid spread of the epidemic were still not well understood. Surveillance systems mainly focused on tracking of AIDS cases and the spread of HIV. But such surveillance only documented the damage that had already been wrought on the individuals, families, communities and the country. This did not help in identifying factors such as current behaviours, which fuel the HIV pandemic. Documenting such behaviours which predispose to the spread of HIV/AIDS was of crucial importance for prevention of the epidemic. We developed a new framework for HIV surveillance to address this information gap. The behavioural surveillance surveys (BSS), aptly called the second-generation surveillance system were based on tracking behavioural changes in the country.

We decided to launch the first BSS soon after commissioning of NACP II, but it took some time to develop the protocols and recruit an agency for conducting the survey. After scouting for expertise we decided to entrust the work to ORG MARG, an independent agency which had conducted such community-based surveys earlier. Salil Panakadan, and G.V.S. Murthy from All India Institute of Medical Sciences (AIIMS), maintained close supervision over the survey and had made midcourse corrections in some states such as Andhra Pradesh. The first survey was undertaken from March to August 2001, in all the 32 states and union territories with more than 85,000 samples drawn from general population. A second round of survey for vulnerable groups was done from October 2001 to March 2002, with 5572 sex workers, 5648 clients, 1355 IDUs and 1387 MSMs interviewed for the survey. Such a large-scale survey for HIV/AIDS was the first of its kind, done under strict quality control and supervision. Several behaviour-related indicators were included in the survey such as awareness of HIV/AIDS, sexually transmitted infections (STIs), condom use, sexual behaviour and exposure to mass media and IEC campaigns. The results indicated high differential across the states in important indicators, for example levels of awareness on HIV/AIDS, STIs, condom use and mother-to-child transmission. Some interesting results which flowed out of the survey were low levels of awareness about STIs even in states with high HIV awareness levels, low level of awareness about the connection between HIV and STIs and on breast-feeding as a cause of vertical transmission. But the most surprising data was on sex with nonregular partners, which is a serious risk factor for heterosexual transmission of HIV. A high proportion of adult males (11.8%) reported having sex with a nonregular partner, while the percentage of females was low at 2% as a national average. More surprising was the high percentage of multipartner sex among males and females in Maharashtra and Andhra Pradesh, two of the high prevalence states at 19 and 7.4 in Andhra Pradesh and 15 and 7.3 in Maharashtra, respectively. The strong correlation with high HIV prevalence among both males and females in these two states couldn't be missed.

But those states were still not showing strong commitment to strengthen the AIDS response. I thought it was necessary to bring the risk factor of sex outside the marriage to the notice of their highest political authorities. We started with Andhra Pradesh; its CM was tech savvy and had introduced computer-based monitoring systems for many state government programmes much earlier than the rest of the country. He gave time to a delegation from NACO and the World Bank where the BSS results were presented. The high percentage of adult men and women who indulge in multipartner sex in Andhra Pradesh surprised its CM. He could sense the serious risk of a runaway AIDS epidemic fueled by unprotected multipartner sex. In the next few months we witnessed several initiatives from him such as positioning full-time senior IAS officials, Chandramouli and Damayanthi, as PDs of SACS, and entrusting monitoring of HIV prevention programmes to the district collectors, the heads of district administration. The CM regularly held video conferences with the district functionaries and AIDS response became an important issue for review. The programme took an upturn and since then Andhra Pradesh joined the states which were in the forefront of HIV response in the country.

Box 1: A Chief Minister Takes the Lead

Majority of Indian population shuns even speaking about HIV/AIDS, but not Chandrababu Naidu, the CM of Andhra Pradesh from 1998 to 2004. 'Indian sentiment is not to talk about sex, so people like me have to talk about it', he says. 'When the predominant mode of transmission of HIV/AIDS happens to be unsafe sexual practices, there is silence on the whole issue. Unless this silence is broken and people talk about HIV/AIDS, it is not possible to stop the silent spread of this dreadful disease. Once I realised this, I made sure that silence is broken'. This is a job that must be led by political leaders to be effective, Naidu insists. 'When a leader talks on these issues, thousands listen and understand its importance. When the leader speaks and calls for action, the cadre responds… This is essential. If the leaders talk, the community talks. Breaking the silence is the first step in the fight against the epidemic'.

Naidu's methods as CM were varied, energetic and sometimes unconventional. He had erected a giant, inflated condom in front of the state assembly to break down public inhibitions about discussing matters related to sex. He made mandatory for the ministers of the state government to include the issue of HIV/AIDS in all their speeches and public meetings. He had also put it firmly on the agenda of the state assembly, ensuring that politicians devoted 1 day of every session to discuss the issue.

'People say to me, "Sir, what about the sanctity of the family"? I say our job is to protect the sanctity of people's lives—human beings—and we have people dying'.

He vigorously promoted life skills education, including reproductive health in schools. When one private school resisted, he ruled that none of its pupils would have their exam results recognised. He had also pushed for condoms to be distributed free wherever alcohol is sold, and at all official functions.[1]

Maharashtra and the city of Mumbai were also in the thick of the epidemic. Right from my first visit to Mumbai in 1997, I was convinced that Mumbai needed a focused response. I suggested to the state government that Mumbai should start a separate AIDS control society with full involvement of the Brihanmumbai Municipal Corporation (BMC; formerly Bombay Municipal Corporation) in its management. Maharashtra was the only state where we operated separate AIDS control societies for the state and for BMC. This had shown good results as senior officials of BMC started taking interest in AIDS programmes and provided leadership to the Mumbai SACS. The state government also positioned senior officers such as Medha Gadgil and Alka Gogte as PDs. The BMC provided a building, formerly an old leprosy hospital in Wadala, Central Mumbai, to accommodate both the Maharashtra and Mumbai AIDS control societies. The building was refurbished and till today is one of the best locations of AIDS control offices.

Constant engagement and person-to-person contact with chief secretaries and health secretaries of states enabled the programme to get senior and dedicated officials to head the SACS. By 2000, majority of the larger and high-burden states placed senior-level government functionaries as PDs and technical heads in the AIDS control societies. I looked at the BSS as an important instrument for generating political will in states which were still lagging behind. Our constant engagement with the state leadership in high prevalence states had lifted the programme to a high level of visibility. Tamil Nadu, which was a forerunner, was the best example of a committed political leadership and bureaucracy, lending support to implementors from civil society as well as government.

In the area of care and support, the Tambaram Hospital in Chennai served as the nodal centre for providing treatment for opportunistic infections and palliative care for AIDS patients, not just from Tamil Nadu and neighbouring states such as Andhra Pradesh and Karnataka, but states as far as West Bengal and Maharashtra. C.N. Deivanayagam, the superintendent of the hospital, was a pioneer with high level of commitment to provide care to AIDS patients. His methods were at times unconventional but his commitment and feel for the infected people drew many patients to the Tambaram hospital. The TRG on care and support was established there, mainly because of the excellent team of health care professionals he could assemble in the centre.

SEX WORKER INTERVENTIONS

Reduction of new infections was our foremost priority, and Component 1 of NACP for prevention interventions (TIs) among most at-risk populations was the key to the success of the programme. Serosurveillance conducted since 1986 had shown that heterosexual transmission accounted for almost 85% of the infections occurring in India.

Sex work–commercial and casual–was the main route of HIV transmission, not just in urban areas but even in the countryside. This was fueled by migrant workers and transport workers whose mobility and propensity for unprotected multipartner sex was the most important risk factor. Major truck routes and halting stations became centres of high prevalence of HIV and AIDS. Places such as Namakkal in Tamil Nadu, Sangli in Maharashtra, Guntur and Rajahmundry in Andhra Pradesh, Bagalkot in Karnataka, became prominent hot spots on the

AIDS map of India. Commercial sex was mostly brothel-based in the 1990s. Street-based and casual sex was just emerging on the scene but brothel-based interventions were still the most effective to control new infections.

But this was an area least familiar to the state societies except one or two like Tamil Nadu and Maharashtra. In West Bengal, Sonagachi was a unique sex worker intervention programme funded directly by DFID. The TI model we developed in-house was based on the Sonagachi model with necessary modifications. We had to put in position an elaborate training programme for SACS officials and NGO Advisors on how to design and implement TIs for groups of sex workers. Sex worker sites were carefully mapped in all states and an open advertisement was issued for NGOs and community-based organisations (CBOs) to apply for grants. A selection committee chaired by the health secretary of the state government was entrusted with the process of finalising the agencies. This open process ensured selection of the best agencies and involvement of the state health administrators in the TI programmes. It was a transformative process for many of the agencies who were functioning earlier as activists and advocates for AIDS programmes to become responsible implementors with accountability for performance and proper utilisation of public funds.

By 2002, we scaled-up the programme to 181 interventions covering a population of 450,000 sex workers. This large coverage of sex workers and their clients effectively led to impressive reduction of infection rates among sex workers by 2010.

Box 2: Sex Workers' Interventions–Sonagachi Project

The 7000 strong brothels in Sonagachi in the city of Kolkata (Calcutta at that time), had the best sex workers' intervention which could serve as a model for scaling-up across the country. A vertical HIV intervention programme was launched in 1992, following a base-line study initiated by NACO in association with GPA WHO and conducted by All India Institute of Hygiene & Public Health (AIIH&PH), a Central Government institute in Kolkata. Smarajit Jana from the institute took the lead in conducting the study and found that more than HIV and STI-related matters, the sex workers were concerned about their infertility problems and desire to have children. These results enabled him and his team to adopt a more humanistic approach towards the sex worker community instead of seeing them as objects of sex. The intervention programme started with the three 'Rs', reliance, respect and recognition and consisted of three principal components: provision of health services including STI treatment; information, education and communication (IEC) and condom programming. The programme was pivoted on 'peer-based approach'. Sex workers recruited from the community were provided training on health and HIV and were promoted as peers and outreach workers. Their role was to spread HIV-related messages among their colleagues and friends and help them avail clinical services in addition to condoms. However, over a period of time, various environmental factors such as police raid, extortion by the local goons, and negative attitude of service providers as well as from a section of researchers limited the reach of the sex workers to access and to utilise preventive services. They started recognising the need for inclusion of empowering strategies to address various structural issues.

In 1995, a unique body of the 'fallen women' Durbar Mahila Samanwaya Committee (DMSC) came into existence. This was a forum exclusively set up and managed by sex workers and their children with the objective of creating solidarity and collective strength among the sex worker community and other marginalised groups.

The project was initially financed by Norwegian Aid Agency (NORAD) in December 1992, and from October 1994 by DFID the British Aid agency, until NACO brought it into the ambit of NACP II in 1999 and started financing the interventions.

DMSC took over the management of STD/HIV intervention programme (SHIP) from AIIH&PH by 1999. After taking the full control of the intervention programme, DMSC started replicating the basic principles and guiding policies of 'Sonagachi Project' in other red light areas of the city. The organisation took special initiative to reach an increasing number of sex workers by promoting agency of the sex workers and putting stress in their collective bargaining power, both in accessing services related to safer sex as well as in improving working condition of sex workers. DMSC claims that for any intervention programme to succeed, it should call for sociopolitical activism with up-to-date knowledge and information, and sound skills and capacity of its staff members.

Economic insecurity coupled with extortionate money lending practices that exist only in red light areas had always been part of the lives of sex workers. They were unable to save their incomes and escape debt traps. To change this, they took one of the most significant steps by registering a consumer cooperative society (Usha Multipurpose Co-operative Society Limited, or Usha). Usha is for and by sex workers. In August 1995, DMSC succeeded in persuading the Government of West Bengal to remove the relevant clauses from the cooperative law to enable registration of the society as the cooperative of 'sex workers' rather than being passed off as ubiquitous 'housewives'. The registration of the cooperative marks an important strategic advantage for sex workers in DMSC's struggle to reframe the definitions and meanings of their occupation. The Cooperative society could enlist 16,000 members for economic support in times of need.[2]

CONDOM PROMOTION

Since inception of the NACP, public provisioning and promotion of condom use were carried out using the existing mechanisms under the Department of Family Welfare (DFW) which was implementing a large programme for free distribution and social marketing of condoms in the country as a population stabilisation measure. India had a large manufacturing capacity for condoms with six manufacturers having a combined manufacturing capacity of 2.5 billion condoms per annum.

During NACP II we worked closely with DFW for procument of condoms needed for free and subsidised segments and supply to the State AIDS Control Societies. Procurement of condoms for NACO doubled within 2 years from 128 million pieces to 230 million from 2002 to 2004 and to about 400 million in 2005. Social marketing of condoms prioritised setting up of retail outlets in underserved and nonconventional areas to ensure easy availability at the time and place where they were needed. Some states, for example Andhra Pradesh and Tamil Nadu, used the fair price shops in the public distribution system to open retail outlets for condoms.

For TIs, NACO preferred to directly supply condoms to intervention sites through the implementing NGOs. Sex worker interventions had an important component of condom availability secured through peer educators drawn from the communities. The success of sex worker TIs in a large measure was due to timely availability and use of condoms promoted by regular awareness campaigns targeting the sex workers and clients.

In some intervention sites, the peer educators faced problems with local police who threatened them with arrests for carrying condoms. We asked the SACS to involve senior police officers at the level of district Superintendents of Police (SP) and get directives issued to field-level staff not to harass the peer educators for carrying condoms. In some districts the SPs issued identity cards to the peer educators with their signatures and local police were quick to comply!

INJECTING DRUG USE IN NORTHEASTERN INDIA

Dealing with HIV infection among IDUs posed enormous challenges. It took me time to understand the complexities of drug use in the country as a whole and particularly in North East (NE) India, where injecting of drugs was quite prevalent by 1997. Pattern of substance abuse in NE India underwent rapid changes in the 1980-90s, which needs some elaboration to understand the complexities of HIV spread in that region. These are provided in Box 3.

Box 3

'The UNODC and Ministry of Social Justice & Empowerment (MSJ&E) Government of India provided detailed documentation of the history of spread of substance use in NE in their publication 'Drug Use in North Eastern States of India'. Chewing betel nuts with the leaves of the betel plant and lime paste, and smoking tobacco, were the two most common traditional forms of substance use in almost all the northeastern states of India. Most of these states also witnessed cannabis smoking, drinking of home-brewed rice beer and a limited use of opium (eating and smoking) in traditional tribal societies. Sipping nicotine water (known as 'tuibuk', 'tuibur' or 'hidakphu' in some places and eating fried vegetable cakes (locally known as 'baras' or 'pakoras') prepared with cannabis leaves as one of the ingredients are two other examples of traditional use of psychotropic substances in this part of the country.

Following the introduction of heroin in NE India during the early 1970s, drug use among the local youths took a new turn. Within ten years' time, heroin smoking – a non-traditional form of opiate use – replaced the traditional use of cannabis and opium to a great extent in some of the states. A fairly large number of heroin smokers subsequently switched to injecting heroin and synthetic pharmaceutical painkillers such as dextropropoxyphene (sold under the trade name Proxyvon® or Spasmoproxyvon®). The major reason for this shift from smoking to injecting is increased tolerance. More money was needed by the long-term heroin smokers for frequent 'chasing' to obtain the same effect that they used to get with lesser amount of heroin during the early days of heroin use. Injecting heroin therefore became a practical solution to this.

The Report truly reveals that widespread concern over drug use in northeast India, however, only followed the outbreak of the HIV epidemic among local heroin injectors in Manipur in October 1989, which then attracted the attention of many national and international communities.[3]

By 1997, considerable data existed about the explosive spread of HIV epidemic in Manipur, Nagaland and Mizoram; three states that share international border with Myanmar. Cross-border trafficking of drugs such as heroin and pharma pain killer dextropropoxyphene had therefore a direct impact on HIV spread in these states. Use of dextropropoxyphene was fairly widespread with drugs such as Spasmo-Proxyvon available easily from medicine shops in NE as cough syrups.

The introduction of amphetamines in late-1990s added a new dimension to drug use in North East. Oral use of amphetamines as a pleasure-enhancing substance became widespread within a very short period of time. Unlike heroin and related drugs which are 'downers' or make the consumer inactive, amphetamines are 'enhancers' which induce the consumer into high-risk unprotected sexual behaviour. The spread of HIV among young female partners of drug users in NE India could partly be ascribed to amphetamine use.

An Indian Council of Medical Research (ICMR) team led by Swarup Sarkar and Samiran Panda in their UNODC publication described the explosive spread of HIV in Manipur 'Manipur has been a classic example of a sharp rise in seroprevalence among injectors within a short span of time. Serosurveillance started in Manipur in 1986, when a total of 2,322 persons, including 707 intravenous drug users, were screened, and the first seropositive intravenous drug user was detected in October 1989. Within two years the percentage of cases tested positive jumped to 60% showing an explosive rise in infection rates among IDUs in Manipur.'[4]

Under the first phase of NACP, limited sentinel surveillance was conducted among IDUs in Manipur and Nagaland, which also reported an explosive HIV epidemic with prevalence levels of 70% in Imphal, 50% in Churachandpur, Manipur, and 25% in Nagaland. The Government of Manipur got alerted by this high prevalence of HIV and brought out a State AIDS Control Policy in 1996 outlining steps to combat the epidemic, the first of its kind for any state in India.

In the first nationwide sentinel survey conducted in 1999, we confirmed higher HIV prevalence among IDUs in Manipur, Nagaland and Mizoram compared to other states in NE. This was ascribed to easy availability of drugs from across the international border with Myanmar. Prevalence of HIV among IDUs was comparatively less at 1.6% in Mizoram in 1999, but shot up to 9.6% by 2000. The number of sentinel sites were 12, still very few compared with the STI and antenatal care (ANC) sites.

We faced challenges in accessing NE states because of the remoteness of areas of drug use and militancy in Manipur. The attitude of mainstream society towards drug users in general was indifferent, bordering on hostility. SACS were established in all NE states that received funding for IDU interventions from NACO. Governance of the SACS and management of programmes was a big challenge as all the states could not deploy senior-level functionaries as PDs.

As opposed to that, the community leadership and active networking of drug user community were great assets for the programme. Many of the NGOs and CBOs were promoted by former and current drug users who had intimate knowledge of the issues and challenges. Even during the NACP I, intervention projects for IDUs funded by Swedish International Development Cooperation Agency (SIDA) were getting implemented by NGOs in Manipur and Nagaland. A network of IDUs called North East India HIV/AIDS Network (NEIHAN) was also supported by SIDA for capacity building. The activities of NEIHAN included the sharing of information, experiences and lessons learnt on HIV/AIDS and drug-use-related interventions through formation of e-groups and the holding of workshops to influence policy change through the regional coalition of stakeholders in NE India. Shortly thereafter the drug user community who were HIV-positive established the Manipur network of HIV-positive people (MNP+), one of the first positive networks established in India.

The TI model adopted for NACP II for IDUs was then applied to interventions in NE. Supply of clean needles under a needle and syringe exchange protocol was an important component of the TI module. Oral substitution with either methadone or buprenorphine was still relatively unknown as an intervention strategy in India. Methadone, a prohibited drug under the Narcotics and Psychotropic Substances Act was not available for intervention programmes. The National AIDS Control Policy 2002 endorsed harm reduction interventions for prevention of HIV among IDUs. Taking advantage of this policy prescription, demonstration projects for needle and syringe exchange were taken up for implementation in West Bengal and Chennai. Sublingual buprenorphine was licensed in India for the treatment of opioid dependence by drug abuse treatment centres since 1999.[4] Needle and syringe exchange programmes were taken up on a large scale and funds were provided to the SACS for supporting NGOs and IDU networks. The number of TIs progressively increased to 77 in the three states of Manipur, Nagaland and Mizoram (NACO report to WB Mission March 2006) out of 93 for the entire country. A coverage estimation of IDUs by TIs done by NACO showed that by the end of NACP II, 88,194 IDUs were covered under the TIs, majority of them in the three northeastern states.[5]

The impact of these prevention programmes was mixed. On the positive side, the explosive growth of HIV in Manipur and Nagaland could be contained. Even though the prevalence levels were higher than in general population at the end of the second phase, the needle and syringe exchange programmes gained acceptability with the drug user community. The massive HIV awareness campaigns taken up in the region with active participation of the positive networks and the drug user community were important contributory factors to the relative stabilisation of the IDU epidemic in Manipur and Nagaland. But the neighbouring state of Mizoram started reporting higher prevalence of HIV among the IDU community with levels touching 9.6% by 2000. Number of interventions was also fewer than in Nagaland and Manipur. Today Mizoram is one of the few states of the country, which is still showing a rise in incidence, beating the national trend of declining infection rates.

The challenge that NACO faced in raising general awareness about drug use and its connection with HIV was to find a platform to launch a campaign for sensitisation of drug user community on their vulnerability to HIV/AIDS. The Ministry of Social Justice and Empowerment (MSJE), an important wing of the government dealing with social sector issues became our partner. MSJE was implementing an important programme for prevention of alcohol and drug abuse in the country since 1986. The activities funded through NGOs included de-addiction/rehabilitation centres (DRCs), counselling centres (CCs) and de-addiction camps. A total of 362 such addiction treatment centres were getting funding from MSJE under this scheme. Based on the recommendations of a workshop NACO organised jointly with UNODC and MSJE, we decided to add an HIV component to the interventions in 100 DRCs by providing funds directly from NACP II as an intersectoral activity. The MSJE responded favourably to this proposal and gave permission for recruiting an additional counsellor/

field worker in each of the centres. Funds were first made available in March 2001. Sharan, a Delhi-based NGO, was commissioned to prepare a training module for imparting training to the staff of the de-addiction centres and the newly recruited counsellors. About 94 centres recruited the counsellors and implemented the programme which was one of the best intersectoral initiatives undertaken by NACO under NACP II. I was keen to know the outcome of this collaboration through an independent evaluation of the partnership to gauge the extent of integration of HIV/AIDS issues into the work of NGOs on drug demand reduction under the collaboration, and to make recommendations for future steps to strengthen and scale-up the collaborative effort. Family Health International (FHI) was asked to conduct the evaluation and present recommendations on the impact for further strengthening the collaborative effort. The evaluation results were presented to NACO in April 2004. The report commended the joint effort of the two government agencies and the uniqueness of the collaborative effort, and made recommendations for its further continuance.

But it was not until 2007 that the first national network of harm reduction advocates could be established with the mission of securing access to quality health services for drug users within a rights-based framework and to support their participation in policy and implementation of programmes. The Indian Harm reduction Network (IHRN) was initiated with 43 members in 2007 of which 15 were service providing NGOs and 28 harm reduction experts and community organisations. The network established 4 regional harm reduction networks–North, South, East and West. NEIHRN for North East was already engaged and provided support including securing technical support and funds from UNAIDS.

MSM AND TRANSGENDER ISSUES

> **Box 4**
>
> 'The term LGBT includes Lesbian, Gay, Bi sexual and Transgender populations and emphasizes a diversity of sexuality and gender identity-based cultures. The letter Q has been added later to refer to anyone who is not a heterosexual and whose identity can be considered as *queer.* The term **LGBTQ** has been recorded since 1996.* Sometimes the letter I is also added to identify *intersex* people to LGBT groups.[6]
>
> In post-independence India, the LGBTQ (lesbian, gay, bi-sexual, transgender and queer) community faced numerous challenges to establish their rights for separate sexual identity and behaviour.
>
> The first known protest for gay rights was held on Aug. 11, 1992, 45 years after India gained independence from British colonialism. An organisation called AIDS Bhedbhav Virodhi Andolan (ABVA) organised the gathering in front of Delhi police headquarters to protest against the rounding up of men from Connaught Place's Central Park on charges of homosexuality. The protest didn't see any desired outcome.
>
> Two years later in 1994, ABVA activists filed a public interest litigation (PIL) in Delhi High Court challenging the constitutionality of Section 377 of Indian Penal Code (IPC). This PIL was the first legal protest and the first attempt to legalize homosexuality in India. In 1991, ABVA published a report titled 'Less than Gay', a citizen's report on the discrimination faced by the community in India. The PIL provided India with its first champion of gay rights, Siddhartha Gautam, a co-founder of ABVA. However, post-Gautam's early and sudden demise, ABVA failed to follow through on the petition and the case was dismissed in 2001'.[7]

The MSM interventions were the most challenging for us. In the 1990s the stigma surrounding male-to-male sex was so high in India that the community was living mostly underground and not willing to be identified. Section 377 of the Indian Penal Code (IPC) made same-sex relations a criminal offence. Section 377 can be traced back to Britain's Buggery Act of 1533 brought by King Henry VIII. According to Justice Nariman, Section 377 was modeled on the said act which prohibited, 'the detestable and abominable offense of buggery (anal intercourse) committed with mankind or beast'. The section which was introduced in 1861 by the British colonial rulers read as follows:

UNNATURAL OFFENCES

377. Unnatural offences–Whoever voluntarily has carnal intercourse against the order of nature with any man, woman or animal, shall be punished with 1*[imprisonment for life]. or with imprisonment of either description for a term which may extent to ten years, and shall also be liable to fine.

Explanation–Penetration is sufficient to constitute the carnal intercourse necessary to the offence described in this section.

While the section contained strict provisions for violation, there were very few instances of anyone getting convicted with a major punishment under this section. But the presence of these provisions in the act effectively criminalised an entire community whose number was put at 2.5 million by the government itself. Activists felt this is a grossly underestimated figure.

The explosive spread of HIV in India among the vulnerable communities reflected in the LGBTQ population, which also showed much higher prevalence levels than in general population. In 1999, when we conducted the first national level sentinel surveillance, there were no separate sites for LGBTQ community for recording prevalence levels. The STI sites were used as a proxy in areas of reported activity of sex workers and of IDUs in NE. The prevalence of HIV among MSM communities was mainly based on reported community figures which clearly showed an abnormal rise in infection rates due to unprotected sex and lack of awareness about HIV/AIDS. The third dimension was the severe stigma attached to same-sex relations not just because of the legal provision under IPC but the prejudiced attitude of mainstream society towards homosexuality and transgender identity.

We didn't wait for formal surveys to launch an intervention programmes for the LGBTQ community. We looked for possible partners and the only visible organisation we identified was Humsafar Trust in Mumbai run by Ashok Row Kavi, the well-known social activist for gay rights. Ashok Kavi was openly living as gay from 1986. In June 1990, he started the first gay magazine in India, *Bombay Dost,* and in 1994, set up the Humsafar Trust as an organisation of gay men and transgender community.

I thought the best entry point for an MSM intervention was to start with Humsafar Trust. Through the Mumbai District AIDS Control Society (MDACS) we initiated the first pilot project for MSM to provide HIV services such as condom distribution, HIV testing and referral to Sion Hospital, Mumbai. In June 1999, Ashok invited me, joint director of IEC Neelam Kapur and Medha Gadgil, the PD of Maharashtra SACS, to visit his centre and inaugurate the facility in Mumbai. It was a totally new experience for all three of us. We were meeting, for the first time, a group of openly living gay persons introduced to us by Ashok. The visit opened our eyes to a new world we were not aware of. We discussed the need for prevention interventions for the MSM community whose numbers were still unknown. The decision to start the first TI for MSM was the right one as in a period of 1 year the centre was able to reach more than 3000 MSM against the target of 1000 given to them. Later it became a sentinel surveillance site for MSM communities.

But getting a critical number of community leaders to Delhi was crucial to understand the extent of HIV/AIDS problem among the community and the broader issue of sexuality and gender relations among them. We called a consultation meeting of about 20 community leaders in the Ashoka Hotel, Delhi. But the hotel refused to provide them accommodation. We secured accommodation by not revealing their identities and arranged the meeting without a banner or poster. The MSM networks in India took shape from that small and invisible event but spread rapidly across the country. After this meeting the number of TIs for MSMs started growing. By 2004, we identified and enlisted 30 community-based MSM organisations implementing TIs programmes in the country.

But the programme had its challenges and setbacks. In March 2001, the Naz Foundation International (NFI) based in the United Kingdom, wanted to open their regional office in Lucknow. NFI was a community organisation led by Shivananda Khan, an MSM activist who supported the communities, particularly in South Asia. The local administration was not happy with NFI functioning from Lucknow. In July 2001, Arif Jafar, the director and two other personnel were arrested by Lucknow police under Section 377 IPC under the charge of promoting homosexuality. When news reached NACO, I called Bachittar Singh, the PD of UPSACS and asked him to intervene with local police to secure their release. I wrote to the Home Secretary of Uttar Pradesh to intervene with the local police to release the office bearers. The event attracted media attention with major national newspapers like *Times of India* prominently reporting the incident. Getting the three persons released on bail was also an uphill task. The judge was adamant and called homosexuality 'a curse on society and the accused can't be allowed to go scot-free'. It was only after senior lawyers from Delhi intervened that Arif and his two colleagues got bail after 47 days of internment!

The incident of Lucknow brought an upsurge of support to the MSM communities and eased the pressure on their movement and ability to organise into groups and networks despite the Damocles' sword of Section 377 hanging on them. Later in 2006 when I was heading the UNAIDS Regional Support Team (RST) in Bangkok, we supported a regional consultation of MSMs in Asia Pacific in Delhi called 'risks and responsibilities'. There was overwhelming response with nearly 200 representatives from Asia Pacific countries attending the meeting. The Ashoka Hotel which refused the permission earlier had opened the gates of hospitality to the community participants! Apart from community representatives and the UN agencies, the conference saw a number of parliamentarians from India and other Asian countries addressing the participants and pledging support to their cause. Within a period of 5 years there was a radical transformation of the ground level situation with intellectuals, writers, celebrities and prominent citizens from mainstream society supporting their cause and appealing to the government to decriminalise the community by repealing Section 377 IPC. The visits of Justice Kirby from Australia and Justice Cameron from South Africa, the two openly living gay community members, to attend the International Policy Makers Conference on HIV/AIDS in May 2002 and their interaction with the community of lawyers and judges in India provided further strength to the movement.

PEOPLE LIVING WITH HIV/AIDS

The most challenging issue we faced during the first few years of implementation was providing care and support to the increasing number of HIV-positive persons. The HIV national estimates published by NACO in 1998 showed that approximately 3 million people were already infected. Many of those who became symptomatic of AIDS-related infections had to be provided basic care and support for treatment of the opportunistic infections (OIs). Low-cost AIDS care component of NACP consisted of important programmes such as provision of treatment for OIs in all government hospitals, operation of community care and support centres by NGOs for treatment of OIs, voluntary counselling and testing programme and prevention of infections among health care providers by adoption of universal infection control measures and provision of drugs for post exposure prophylaxis (PEP). NGOs established 85 Community Care Centres (CCC) directly funded by NACO as model centres for low-cost AIDS care. Funds were provided to SACS to procure drugs for PEP for protection of health care personnel. Needle-stick injuries were very few and were promptly covered by PEP.

Taking the Thailand example as a model, we started promoting organisations of HIV+ people at national and state level. These efforts were complimented by opening of drop-in centres to promote positive living, to build capacity and to empower PLHAs to protect and promote their rights. Seventy drop-in centres were established and funded by NACO in NACP II which laid the foundation for expansion of positive networks in each state which were federated into a national network. A women's positive network was also started by Kousalya, an enterprising and outspoken HIV+ woman from Tamil Nadu. The spread of HIV+ networks across the country facilitated the empowerment of many HIV+ men and women who took courage to reveal their HIV status and assume leadership of the community. Ashok Pillai, Ramesh Venkataraman, Thoku Yepthomi, Kousalya, Anandi Yuvraj, Celena D'Costa and Jahnabi Goswami were all leaders who availed the opportunity of forming HIV+ networks to provide leadership to the AIDS movement at various points of time during the project period.

I had the personal experience of meeting Jahnabi Goswami while visiting Assam SACS in March 2000. I saw her handling the reception desk of the SACS office and in considerable distress. Dr. Deuri, the PD SACS, informed me that her husband who was a businessman had died of AIDS at a young age and she was facing financial and social challenges with the family of the husband. Deuri appointed her as a receptionist in the office on a temporary basis to provide some financial support. After talking to her I thought she would be suitable to play the role of a counsellor and facilitate networking with other HIV+ persons. She was trained as a counsellor and appointed in the SACS office. Since then Jahnabi discovered herself and in May 2000 delivered her public speech in front of NACO and UN officials on her life and experiences as a person openly living with HIV. She later became the president of the HIV+ network and an outspoken voice for the community. There were many such examples of HIV+ men and women who overcame AIDS-related stigma and assumed leadership of the community.

COUNSELLING AND TESTING FOR HIV

At this stage we also decided to expand testing facilities, not just at the blood banks, but in the community as well. The concept of voluntary testing with pre- and post-test counselling took shape during this period with ease of testing by rapid tests firmly established under the programme. We decided that every district hospital should have a voluntary counselling and testing centre (VCTC) available for general public apart from functioning as a referral centre for the hospital. The first VCTC was established in Ram Manohar Lohia (RML) Hospital Delhi, and within the next 3 years there was a massive scale-up of VCTC facilities across the country. By December 2004, the country had 738 functioning VCTCs operating in 576 districts out of 603. From almost zero the number of walk-in clients seeking voluntary testing had shot up to 30% of the case load within 3 years; the rest 70% were getting referred to from hospitals. Pre- and post-test counselling was provided by trained counsellors who were recruited in large number from CBOs and NGOs. The demand from these centres was so huge that we had started planning to reach to the sub-district level in the next phase of the programme and introduce community-based VCTCs run by NGOs and CBOs. The World Bank Implementation Completion Report (ICR) mentioned that by December 2005 the number of VCTCs shot up to 1114 with 376 centres established in 2005 alone. The phenomenal rise in the awareness levels and health-seeking behaviour of people at large on HIV/AIDS was largely ascribed to this vast network of VCTCs established across the country.

After 20 years, I can confidently say that the 23% programme money we spent on controlling the epidemic among the key populations was the single contributory factor for preventing a runaway HIV epidemic in India and saving the country from the dubious distinction of being named as the AIDS capital of the world. Working closely with all the three at-risk groups–sex workers, IDUs and MSM communities, and people living with HIV/AIDS, standing by their side and taking up their cause on crucial issues provided an identity to NACO as an AIDS advocate, activist and implementor of one of the largest AIDS programmes in the world. The organisation acquired a brand image which was recognisable not just in India but internationally. We designed our own logo when the IEC wing did not find a suitable one on inviting quotations. A website, one of the firsts for any government agency in late 1990s was created and news about the programme were regularly posted and updated. A national helpline number, 1097, was made functional for people seeking information about testing and other facilities available under NACP II.

The ICR of the World Bank, the main lender agency for NACP II certified that by 2005, the overall HIV prevalence among high-risk groups which the programme targeted were brought down to 8.5% in SWs, 5.6% in STI clinic attendants, 10.16% in IDUs and 8.7% in MSM, with great variations.

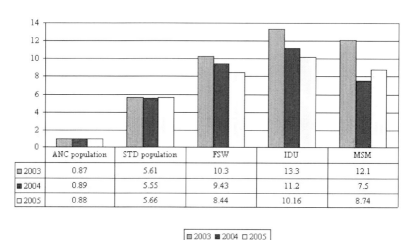

	ANC population	STD population	FSW	IDU	MSM
▨ 2003	0.87	5.61	10.3	13.3	12.1
▪ 2004	0.89	5.55	9.43	11.2	7.5
☐ 2005	0.88	5.66	8.44	10.16	8.74

▨ 2003 ▪ 2004 ☐ 2005

Figure 1: *Annual HIV prevalence rates among various population groups in India (2003-2005). Source: Implementation Completion report NACP II–World Bank March 2006.*

LEGAL ENVIRONMENT

The legal environment for the key populations, however, continued to remain adverse. India had no existing anti-discrimination legislation which would cover discrimination on the grounds of HIV. All the existing laws governing sex work, same-sex relations and drug use criminalised the groups that need to be empowered to access services for prevention care and support under the national programme. The large private sector which provided more than 60% of health services in India did not come under the ambit of any legislation which obligated them to protect the right to health services of the key communities and HIV-positive persons. India was also bound by commitments entered in international agreements and UN covenants which require a review of legal environment surrounding the key populations.

In 1998, I met Anand Grover, a human rights lawyer from Mumbai and was briefed about the activities of his NGO, Lawyers' Collective, in Mumbai. 'The Lawyers Collective HIV/AIDS Unit was set up in 1981, based on a realization that law, policy and judicial action, that upheld the human rights framework, had a central role to play in effectively dealing with the spread of the HIV epidemic. The Unit's aim of crafting a just, rational and non-discriminatory response to HIV was sought to be furthered by policy level advocacy and research, legal-aid services to people living with HIV and public interest litigation on issues pertaining to HIV'.[8]

The NGO was implementing a programme on providing legal support to HIV-positive persons with a small grant from the European Commission. Anand assembled a group of young lawyers and interns to support him in contesting cases of discrimination against HIV-positive persons and termination of employment of HIV-positive employees. We considered that a separate legislation concerning HIV/AIDS issues was required as the existing laws and policies made it difficult for people living with HIV and marginalised communities to seek redress in law courts. Prime examples were criminalisation of soliciting for sex work, drug use and same-sex relations. We decided to work together on preparation of a comprehensive legislation to protect the rights of HIV-positive persons for access to services provided under the national programme and to ensure protection against discriminatory practices at workplace including employment and at educational institutions. The process of drafting the HIV/AIDS Bill started with the International Policy Makers Conference on HIV/AIDS, held in May 2002 in New Delhi. We set up an Advisory Working Group (AWG), chaired by the NACO to initiate this process. The group consisted of members from civil society and organisations of people living with HIV. On the request of the AWG the Lawyers Collective HIV/AIDS unit agreed to undertook the task of preparing a draft bill on HIV.

The AWG met 12 times between June 2002 and August 2003, to discuss various issues related to the draft law and reviewed the material and literature collected for preparing the draft legislation. I was regularly following up with Anand and his team for an appraisal of the draft; the last time in November 2003 after I joined as the Health Secretary.

But the HIV legislation had a chequered history after that. In April 2017, the legislation finally got approval after several attempts were made by NACO to assemble the final draft; 14 years after it was initially contemplated! The act came into effect from September 2018 after rules and regulations for implementation were notified. I shall discuss more about it in the later chapters.

BLOOD SAFETY AND GENERAL AWARENESS PROGRAMMES

We gave equal importance to general awareness programmes under Component 1. Blood-borne infections accounted for 8% of national prevalence, and cleaning up blood transfusion system was essential. The National Blood Transfusion Council and State Councils were strengthened and regular meetings of the council were held. Mandatory testing of blood was enforced by restructuring the procurement systems and ensuring timely supply of test kits for HIV and hepatitis (Hep) B. Earlier, testing for HIV was being carried out with conventional methods of Eliza and Western Blot which were slow and time-consuming. In 2000, WHO announced a new protocol for testing of blood with rapid tests that gave results same day. Testing policy had to be modified to accommodate rapid tests and the TRG on testing did commendable work in revising the testing guidelines to include rapid tests. When we initiated the national level procurement of about 3 million test kits every year, prices came tumbling down and we procured test kits without any increase in allocation of funds under this component.

The northeastern states started reporting high incidence of Hepatitis C among IDUs as a coinfection to HIV. In some sites of Manipur, the rates were alarming at more than 30%. I thought we must introduce mandatory testing for Hep C also to ensure safe blood, free of both Hep B and C. The cost of Hep C test kits was very high and the procurement cost was considered as prohibitive. We decided to go ahead and floated an international tender for Hep C test kit procurement. We got a surprisingly low offer in view of the large number of kits we had decided to procure. The World Bank and the technical team had also agreed to my proposal to include Hep C testing, which since then became a part of blood safety programme.

Procedures were streamlined for licensing of new blood banks, phasing out of small and uneconomical blood banks, starting of blood component separation facilities in 42 different locations and total ban on professional blood donations. Eight state-of-the art blood banks with large capacity of 50,000 units per annum were planned to be established in underserved areas of the country.

General awareness levels about HIV/AIDS were low in the country when NACP II was launched, and IEC programmes carried out in conventional mode were not effective. We banked upon two large programmes during the Phase II for spreading awareness accompanied by behavioural change in large sections of population, especially young people. We gave priority to the school education programmes and decided to universalise them. Ministries of Education and Youth Affairs were key partners in implementation of school education programmes and the University Talk AIDS (UTA) programmes which went beyond HIV/AIDS and encompassed the entire spectrum of issues on sex and sexuality, drug abuse, relationships and marital ties. The school education programmes were developed with close involvement of the state governments and the UNICEF. The latter worked with the IEC division of NACO and developed an educational module for school children of adolescent age. The programme was named 'Family Life Education Programmes' instead of sex education to avoid opposition from conservative sections who were not in favour of imparting any form of sex education for children. The module was tested in regional workshops with state government representatives and launched in a nationwide campaign. Most of the states could successfully adopt the Family Life Education Programmes into school timetables without affecting the main curriculum.

I travelled to some schools and observed that adolescent boys and girls were listening intently to the lessons on sex education and the process of growing up without any embarrassment.

By the end of NACP II, 76% schools out of 144,409 government secondary and senior secondary schools in the country were covered under the school education programme and 152,000 teachers were trained. Of the 109,750 schools covered during project period, 74,292 were covered with the supported from the World Bank funds while 35,458 were covered from DFID funds. A village talk AIDS programme was launched in 410 districts through Nehru Yuvak Kendras, organisations of youth promoted by the department of Youth Welfare for sensitising out-of-school youth in rural areas, which is a large vulnerable group in India.

FAMILY HEALTH AWARENESS CAMPAIGNS (FHAC)

All along, the general health system stayed away from the largest disease-control programme of the country. Except treating AIDS patients who were admitted with serious illnesses, and running some counselling and testing centres, the public sector hospitals were quite disconnected with the AIDS programme. This was more pronounced at the primary health care level. The vast network of Primary Health Centres (PHC) and Community Health Centres (CHC) which were part of the rural health infrastructure were not involved in prevention programmes. I thought that the best way to spread awareness and bring in behavioural change was to bring in large-scale involvement of the PHC infrastructure through awareness campaigns for the rural men and women of reproductive age. After consultation with my colleagues in NACO and some of the health secretaries of the states, we decided to launch a mass awareness programme in campaign mode throughout the country. Named as Family Health Awareness Campaign (FHAC) the programme aimed at bringing the rural adults, men and women of reproductive age, to the PHCs and CHCs for a fortnight in a carefully organised campaign mode once in a year and provide them treatment for STIs and reproductive tract infections (RTIs) and testing facilities for HIV if they ask. Counsellors were mobilised at campaign centres to provide advice to people who practice high-risk behaviour and counsel them to get tested.

The campaigns received enthusiastic response from the rural population and the health care providers. Health secretaries of many states especially from the low HIV prevalence states of northern India lent strong support to the FHAC. Campaigns were held regularly from 2000 to 2004. The campaigns helped in spreading awareness and health-seeking behaviour about STIs and HIV among the rural adults. But the World Bank, the main funding agency for NACP II, was not enthusiastic about the programme. The cost implications of the programme were their main concern, but the spread and impact were not carefully evaluated. After I left NACO in 2002, the campaigns were not conducted regularly and no evaluation of their impact was done. Some research studies conducted by independent researchers supported the programme design and recommended securing greater involvement of SACS and the health departments of the state governments to make it a success. The strategy to follow the STI/RTI awareness route to generate awareness about HIV/AIDS was appreciated in the reviews. It was therefore not clear why the FHAC was stopped midway during implementation. But the ICR of the World Bank states 'The results and contributions of these campaigns to the development objective of the project were not assessed, and action was not taken by Bank to halt or strengthen the campaigns, which were held regularly for several years'. It was a case of missed opportunity for spreading mass awareness on AIDS and involvement of health care functionaries in prevention of HIV and care and support for infected persons. The campaigns would have provided a smooth pathway for transitioning ART and prevention of mother-to-child transmission (PMTCT) programmes from NACO into the general health care system of the country.

INTERMINISTERIAL COORDINATION

Thanks to the leadership provided by the PM and the parliamentary forum on AIDS, we were able to bring in number of ministries and non-health organisations as partners in the AIDS programme. Prominent among them were the Ministries of Education, Youth Services, Labour and Employment, paramilitary organisations under the Home Ministry, Indian Railways, Steel and Coal Industries and the Defence Services. They were involved from the stage of project preparation and developed their own programme components to be funded under the project. Prevention of HIV spread among the employees of these organisations was the main thrust with emphasis on spreading awareness, ensuring safe blood, providing counselling and testing facilities and low-cost care and support to those who were already infected. The organisations were asked to issue policy directives, emphasising protection of employment of infected persons and ensuring that they were not stigmatised or discriminated at the workplace.

The intersectoral component of NACP II opened many doors for us to spread the message of HIV prevention beyond the mandate of Ministry of Health. An interesting incident had occurred when I went to visit the Employees State Insurance (ESI) Corporation in the Labour Ministry, to meet my service colleague Dinesh Gupta, the Director General (DG) who invited me to speak to his Board and senior management on HIV prevention. When I reached the corporation office the board meeting was on and I was waiting in his room to be called when the topic on AIDS was taken up for discussion. After a while a person came out of the meeting room and asked Gupta's secretary *Arey woh AIDS wala kahan hai?*(where is that AIDS guy?) I came out and said 'I am the AIDS wala'. He was taken aback and said, 'sorry sir, the DG asked you to join the meeting'. I narrated the incident to my colleagues in NACO and we all had a hearty laugh. Since then we used to call ourselves the AIDS messengers or *AIDS walas* in Delhi terminology!

These intersectoral programmes ensured that the main thrust of PM's message that HIV is not merely a health issue but an overall development challenge had effectively reached a young large, and economically productive population of the country.

DEVELOPMENTS ON THE GLOBAL FRONT

UN General Assembly Special Session (UNGASS) 2001

We must make people everywhere understand that the AIDS crisis is not over; that this is not about a few foreign countries, far away. This is a threat to an entire generation; this is a threat to an entire civilization....the General Assembly Special Session will provide us with an occasion as never before to face up to our responsibility to future generations, and take decisive action now to turn back the progress of this terrible disease.

– Kofi Annan, Secretary-General, United Nations

As the implementation of NACP II was in full swing, events on the global front were also moving quickly. The International AIDS Conference 2000 held in Durban, South Africa, had attracted global attention to the tragedy that was unfolding in many sub-Saharan African countries including the host country with HIV prevalence reaching hyper epidemic levels and AIDS-related mortality shooting to alarming rates. We took a delegation of civil society partners, donor representatives and NACO officials to see the AIDS situation in South Africa, and understand what could happen to India if we don't act in time. The CPA of UNAIDS India, Gordon Alexander, facilitated the visit and joined us in the delegation. We were given good support by Olavi Elo, the Director of Country Programmes and Swarup Sarkar from UNAIDS. I joined a meeting of countries with large populations which can potentially have a high-disease burden if HIV was not checked in time.

The Conference witnessed large and angry protests by civil society participants at the virtual inaction of governments in the region to the plight of people and families affected by HIV/AIDS. On the political front a battle was on between President Thobo Mbeki of South Africa and the global scientific community which was aghast at the strange logic of Mbeki that HIV does not cause AIDS. He argued that it was poverty and not HIV, which was the most important reason for AIDS spread and deaths in South Africa. A group of 5000 scientists and public health experts signed what was famously known as 'Durban Declaration' affirming that HIV indeed is the cause for AIDS. Even though it was written several weeks before the Durban Conference, it was published a few days before the inauguration of the event in the medical journal *Nature*.[9] The declaration called the evidence that HIV causes AIDS 'clear-cut, exhaustive and unambiguous.'

Undeterred by the criticism, President Mbeki called on scientists to have 'sufficient tolerance to respect everybody's point of view.' Mbeki used his opening address to the conference to compare the campaign against AIDS with the struggle against apartheid. This was promptly countered by the chair of the conference, Jerry Covadia, that HIV was the main cause of AIDS. Poverty only exacerbated HIV/AIDS but was not its basic cause. But the strongest rebuttal came from Justice Edwin Cameron, the South African High Court Judge openly living with HIV who criticised the South African Government for 'mismanaging the epidemic almost at every conceivable turn'. I was among those thousands who assembled to hear Justice Cameron speaking in an open and forthright manner and applauded him. I met him a couple of times after that conference, the last in 2012 as a member of the Global Commission on HIV and Law.

The message of the global community was heard across the world, leading to another important landmark in the fight against AIDS. Within weeks after the Durban Conference the UN Security Council passed a resolution recognising the considerable threat that HIV/AIDS posed to international and regional stability and security. The resolution called for additional actions 'among relevant United Nations bodies, Member States, industry, and other relevant organizations' to discuss issues on HIV/AIDS prevention and care.[10] In the September 2000 Millennium Summit, the General Assembly resolved to keep 'halting and reversing the HIV/AIDS epidemic by 2015' as a Millennium Development Goal (MDG) and voted to hold an emergency special session to address the problem of HIV/AIDS.

In normal course a Special Session of UN General Assembly will need at least a year to two of preparation. But considering the urgency of the problem, the process was fast-tracked. In 2001, two informal consultations were held in quick succession from February 26 to March 2 and from May 21 to May 25, at UN Headquarters, New York. I was invited to participate in the consultations as head of NACO. I met several leading AIDS activists, national programme chiefs, Peter and his colleagues from UNAIDS. The delegates highlighted AIDS-related stigma, protection of human rights, access to prevention and ART services, women's rights to health including reproductive health as areas of outstanding priority.

The UN General Assembly Special Session (UNGASS) was held from 25 to 28 June 2001, with strong representation from the Heads of States and Heads of Governments from Africa, Caribbean and countries of the developed world. In a break from the past, the General Assembly asked national governments to include members of civil society and people living with HIV and their organisations in their country delegations. More than 900 civil society representatives participated in the Special Session, which was quite unprecedented.

The composition of the Indian delegation posed problems as PM Vajpayee was not available due to indisposition. The question of who will head the Indian delegation was very much on our minds. We were surprised when the PMO informed us that the PM nominated Mrs. Sonia Gandhi, the leader of the Opposition in the Lok Sabha, the lower house of parliament to lead the delegation. This was quite unexpected but we all could sense the message PM Vajpayee was trying to convey to the global body about the Indian democratic system and its values. We organised briefing sessions for Mrs. Gandhi in New Delhi and later in New York. On the appointed day she delivered her address in the General Assembly calling for immediate action for preventing the spread of the epidemic and for saving millions of lives by providing treatment support. She appealed to the developed world to come forward with liberal aid to prevent a global tragedy. A leader of the opposition heading the Indian delegation was greatly appreciated by many member country representatives. Some of them came to our seats in the assembly hall and congratulated us.

All through the 3 days of deliberations we could notice the strong presence of UN Secretary-General, Kofi Annan, who was the moving force behind the session. But the negotiations were tortuous and continued until late night on all days. While there was general support and agreement on scaling-up financial resources for HIV prevention and treatment programmes, the controversial parts were on reproductive rights of women to which some countries in the Islamic block objected. The U.S. Government took a different stand compared to the rest of the developed world in its strategy for prevention, laying greater stress on abstinence and being faithful and keeping contraceptive use only as the third alternative. This had surprised many as the general expectation was that United States would lead the developed world in advocating an aggressive strategy to stem the tide of the epidemic.

The statement of commitment which was finally adopted on the last day was one of the strongest assertions of the global community's resolve to take the battle headlong instead of finding soft solutions. Developed countries were asked to provide resources not just for AIDS programmes but for supporting the health and development budgets of developing world by committing 0.7% of their gross domestic product (GDP). Specially on HIV/AIDS, the declaration called for annual commitment of $7 to 10 billion which was quite unprecedented. The declaration called for setting up a global fund for HIV/AIDS to channelise resources for AIDS programmes. Right to Health was recognised as a basic human right and was linked with other civil and political rights, which was also a great improvement on other human rights conventions.

But some CSOs were disappointed with the lack of emphasis on reproductive rights in the declaration. 'While the Declaration generally recognised the important links between human rights and health, especially in the context of HIV/AIDS, it failed to include the term "reproductive rights", or to otherwise reaffirm a comprehensive approach to addressing the right to sexual and reproductive health and self-determination, as was advocated in previous international instruments'.[11]

Around the same time, back in India a momentous announcement shook the pharmaceutical world. Yusuf Hamied, the head of pharmaceutical firm CIPLA, announced a drastic reduction of the prices of first-generation ARV drugs.

Until 2001, ART used to cost $12,000 to $15,000 per patient per year. Hamied combined three ARVs into a single pill called 'triomune', making it easier and more effective for patients to take and offered it at the rate of $350 a patient a year. His announcement caused acute anxiety for the drug multinationals who called him a 'pirate' for offering a generic version of a combination of three patented medicines. But Hamied had evoked great excitement and hope among AIDS patients and their support groups around the world. To them he was a Robin Hood.

In 2001, only 4000 Africans could afford the high-priced branded products. The number got multiplied several times and as per UNAIDS estimates, currently about 20 million HIV-positive persons are accessing

ART and leading normal lives. The cost of first-generation ARVs came down further to around $85 per patient per year.

GLOBAL FUND ON AIDS, TUBERCULOSIS AND MALARIA (GFATM)

The high level of optimism at the close of the UNGASS was sustained by the announcement of a transitional process for constitution of a Global Fund on HIV/AIDS. A Transitional Working Group (TWG) was established in July 2001, with Minister of Health Crispus Coyonga from Uganda as Chair, and included nearly 40 representatives of developing countries, donor countries, NGOs, the private sector and the United Nations system. I represented India on the TWG and attended the group meetings held thrice in quick succession in 2001 in Brussels. In addition, the TWG held regional consultations in Africa, Asia, Latin America and Eastern Europe, as well as thematic consultations with NGOs/civil society, the private sector and academia.

The group developed basic guidelines for the Global Fund's operation, including its legal status, management structure, financial systems and general eligibility criteria. The group in its final report to the UNSG recommended that the Global Fund should be set up for the elimination of AIDS, tuberculosis (TB) and malaria with Headquarters at Geneva administered by a Board and its subcommittees. It will be supported by a technical resource panel for examining and recommending funding proposals from countries. The World Bank would act as the trustee for holding the funds.

The Global Fund came into existence as an international financing institution and was initially recognised as a Swiss foundation on 22 January 2002. On 13 December 2004, the Swiss Federal Council accorded the Global Fund an international organisation status and related privileges and immunities. The developing countries were represented on the board as members of their regional groupings. The United States got elected as the board chair and Thailand as the vice chair of the board from South East Asia Region.

The Global Fund did not go for field offices in implementing countries. A three-level country structure was evolved to manage and monitor implementation of programmes. A Country Coordinating Mechanism (CCM), a partnership composed of key stakeholders in a country's response to the three diseases was made responsible for submitting funding requests to the Global Fund, nominating prospective recipients of Global Fund grants and overseeing grant implementation. The principal recipient (PR), designated by the CCM, would be the recipient of Global Fund financing and utilises it to implement programmes, either directly or through other organisations (sub-recipients). The local fund agent (LFA) would be a key external service provider responsible for monitoring and verifying in-country grant implementation and providing recommendations to the secretariat on key decisions relating to grants.

In India we have established the CCM in 2002 and got the LFA appointed for monitoring the programmes. When we were getting ready for preparing proposals in round 1 for funding from NACO, I got my promotion to the rank of a Secretary to Government in August 2001. A number of officers from my batch in IAS were also promoted around the same time and the government was busy finding ministries where we could be posted as secretaries. I was happy that finally I reached the topmost rung of civil service positions in the GOI, but was not in a mood to leave the national AIDS control efforts in the middle. The programme picked up momentum and we were achieving all round progress. I very much wanted to continue my role as the head of the programme for some more time. Therefore when the government wanted me to continue in NACO but with the rank of a special secretary, until they appointed me in a regular position, I readily agreed. A special secretary gets the same rank and scale of secretary but will not be in charge of a full-fledged department or ministry. I had no problem in working under the overall guidance and supervision of Javid Chowdhury, the Health Secretary, with whom I shared a warm and friendly relationship. He was happy with my contributions in NACO and wanted me to spend more time with other works in the ministry as he felt that NACO was cruising well and did not need my full-time attention. But I did not want the programme to slow down due to lack of attention. I had a hard time shuttling between Nirman Bhavan and Chandralok building, sharing my time and meeting the steadily increasing needs of the Ministry of Health in its regulatory and development functions. This was one of the busiest periods of my stay in the ministry, but it helped me to get prepared for the higher responsibility of secretary a year later.

During this period I was working closely with Javid Chowdhury in formulating a new National Health Policy. The health policy was not revised or updated after the last policy document was issued in 1983, and this vacuum had created problems in addressing health priorities in the fast-changing scenario. The 1983 Policy did not address the critical issue of resource requirement for health. The public spending on health in India was still very low, around 1% of GDP and there was no clear definition of what should be the optimum resource base to address the minimum health needs of the people. Getting associated with the preparation process consumed lot of my time but I saw this as an opportunity to get the national AIDS control policy also approved. The AIDS control policy reached its final stages of preparation after widespread consultations with state governments, CSOs, other ministries and departments in the government and most importantly– the communities of key populations and HIV-positive persons. The Blood Policy also got ready and we decided to announce it as an annex to the AIDS Policy. Finally the Union Cabinet gave approval to the National AIDS Prevention and Control Policy in 2002. Soon after, we got the approval for the new National Health Policy in 2002, just before Javid Chowdhury retired as the Health Secretary.

STINT IN FAMILY WELFARE

Life is full of surprises. When I was expecting that I would succeed Javid as the Health Secretary, I was asked by the government to take charge of the sister department of Family Welfare (FW) as Secretary. Health and Family Welfare were the two important wings of the Ministry of Health headed by two secretaries. They remained as separate departments of Ministry of Health until 2005 when they were merged into a single department of Health & Family Welfare. The FW department dealt with the large health care infrastructure in the country at the primary level and provided funding support to state governments under number of centrally sponsored schemes for primary health care, reproductive health, immunisation and population stabilisation. Eradication of polio was a major programme under the FW department. Providing funding support to sub-centres, the lowest level of health care infrastructure in the country and building their capacity to provide preventive health services was an important function of the department. After long 5 years of association with NACO I finally handed over the charge and joined as Secretary FW in June 2002.

While I got busy addressing all these exciting national priorities, I was missing my work in NACO and NACP II and all the civil society linkages we carefully established over the past 5 years. Even while attending to DFW work I was following the developments connected with the implementation of NACP II. I was disturbed to hear that the Ministry of Information decided to ban TV advertisements on condom use, which were a part of the IEC campaign started by NACO. An organisation called the Joint Action Front for Women complained to the PM and Information and Broadcasting (I&B) Minister that the condom promotion campaigns devised by NACO and Prasar Bharati Corporation, the public broadcaster, were disempowering for women, promoting promiscuity and encouraging violence. The group claimed that condom was not a prescription for AIDS control! The Information Ministry's viewpoint was that condom advertisements should only focus on sex with husband instead of on safe sex. The emphasis was on abstinence and being faithful to husband and use condoms. This was strikingly similar to the ABC campaign advocated by President George Bush in United States, around the same time. NACO promptly shifted its entire condom promotion strategy to the ABC approach. In United States, institutions that promote public health standards such as the National Institutions of Health (NIH) and the Centers for Disease Control and Prevention (CDC) agreed that 'providing complete and accurate information to adolescents about proper use of condoms to reduce the risk of HIV transmission is an essential part of the limited anti HIV arsenal'.[12] The programmes were devised after a lot of research into their usefulness in bringing behaviour change among adult viewers but the government thought they were not suitable for child viewing. I felt that NACO should have effectively contested this decision. I was sure that we were losing an important component in our IEC campaign to spread the message of safe sex to young adults and adolescents, not just for the prevention of HIV but for unsafe sex in marriage and family planning.

Unexpectedly in a cabinet reshuffle, Sushma Swaraj, a senior leader in the ruling National Democratic Alliance (NDA) heading the Information Ministry was posted as the new Cabinet Minister for Health in January 2003. She had lost the Information Ministry, but retained the portfolio of Minister of Parliamentary Affairs as additional charge. The first issue she had to encounter with the media was the ban on condom advertisements and whether she would review the policy as the new health minister. She emphatically replied that her views would continue to be the same. She felt that unsafe sex was not the only cause for the spread of AIDS. I was the Secretary FW and NACO was not my direct concern. But on my seeking, she allowed a discussion on why she thought condom advertisements should not be shown on the public broadcasting platforms. She felt that visual media such as TV, which can be accessed by children of all ages, should not show material which was difficult for the child to absorb and follow. For parents of small children who are curious, it would be hard to explain the meaning of the condom advertisement and the underlying message. The policy continued until 2004, when the new government which was voted to power in May 2004 finally lifted the ban on condom advertisements.

But the arrival of a political heavyweight like Sushma Swaraj in the Ministry of Health was otherwise a positive development. The Ministry suffered the maximum due to the political instability that prevailed since the time I had joined NACO. Between 1997 and 2004, when I finally left, six health ministers had entered and exited and Minister Swaraj was the seventh. At the administrative level the same uncertainty continued with six health secretaries changing jobs before me. In the middle of all these changes I was fortunate to get an uninterrupted stint of 7 years in the Ministry of Health, first as Additional Secretary and later as Secretary to provide continuity at senior administrative level.

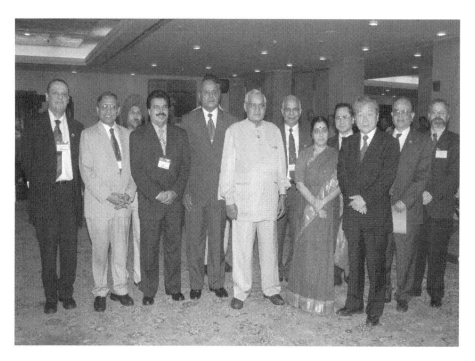

With PM Vajpayee, Minister Sushma Swaraj and DG WHO J.W. Lee

TAKING CHARGE OF HEALTH PORTFOLIO

I developed good working relationship with Minister Sushma Swaraj, who was very quick in understanding the priorities and the relationship between the two departments. She could sense that I was feeling upset for not getting charge of the Department of Health in spite of working as Additional Secretary and Special Secretary for 5 years. When the incumbent secretary finally retired in May 2003, the government had appointed me as Secretary Health. I was sure that Sushma Swaraj played an important role in the shift. I got back the oversight work of NACO and became the Chair of the NACB, the board of management of NACO and the Chair of the Global Fund CCM for India.

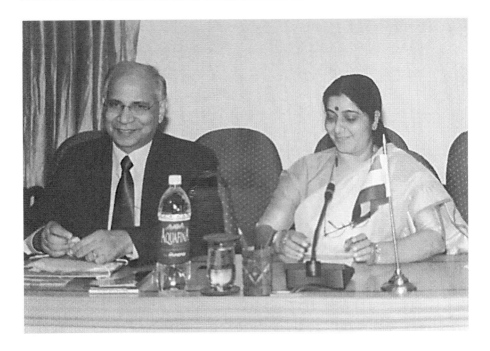

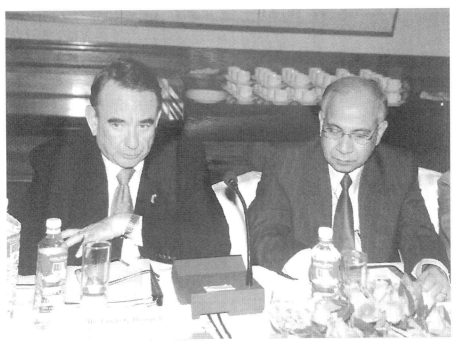

With Minister Sushma Swaraj and US Secretary Health & Human Services, Tommy G.Thompson, at a US mission to Delhi in April 2004.

But being in charge of the programme as PD was entirely different from overseeing it as the head of the department. There was overall concern about the pace of expenditure which was showing signs of slowdown. The project was not able to absorb funds as provided in the project document and the World Bank and other donors were feeling concerned. The project was scheduled to end by 2004, but the signs were evident that it might need an extension.

ANTIRETROVIRAL TREATMENT (ART) PROGRAMME

More important were the civil society voices which were getting shrill because of the non-availability of ART to the growing number of AIDS patients in the country. It was already 2 years since the UNGASS was held and the prices of ARVs plummeted at global level after CIPLA slashed the prices of first-line generic ARVs. In April 2002, WHO added 10 ARV drugs to its list of 'Essential Medicines' and for the first time approved number of generic ARV drugs. In September 2003, WHO declared lack of access to ART as a 'Global Health Emergency' and announced a plan to scale-up access to ARV. The popular '3 by 5' initiative of WHO/UNAIDS launched in December 2003, announced for provision of free ART to 3 million people by end 2005 in developing countries. But the NACP II did not provide any budgetary allocation for ART as the prices were reigning high when the project was being formulated. If ART had to be introduced it should be entirely from domestic budget and no provision existed in the Budget of 2003-2004 for ART.

But Minister Sushma Swaraj was not a person to be deterred by budgetary constraints for decision-making. On 1 December 2003, in a World AIDS Day function she sprang a surprise by announcing that the government had decided to extend ART to all patients whose CD 4 levels were below 250 and to start with, about 17,000 persons would be covered under the programme. I was present in the function and was genuinely surprised as this was never discussed with me before. While leaving the meeting, she smiled and said 'I have made the announcement. And now you people have to make it happen!'

There was great excitement after the announcement but the proof of the pudding was in eating. We had to make it happen. There was hardly any preparation. No formal training was conducted to health care functionaries on ART administration. Drug procurement needed to be put in position and supply chain had to be established. The prices of first-line ARVs were down to almost a dollar a day and the Clinton Foundation, which was already in India, was trying to negotiate a price deal with the generic manufacturers in Maharashtra and Andhra Pradesh.

The health minister asked me to call the manufacturers and arrange a negotiated price for the three-drug combinations of stuvidine, lamvudine and nevirapine. Time was ripe to go for an impactful launch of ART in India.

I called a meeting with generic manufacturers of ARVs and asked them to offer the best prices for India's ART programme; certainly better and more affordable that what they had quoted for Clinton Foundation and others. As the financial year 2003-2004 was closing in a couple of months there was no substantial additional financial liability for that year, but full financial provision had to be made for the next year from domestic resources. The World Bank did not agree to renegotiate the loan and preferred to do it in NACP III, which was already under contemplation. The Planning Commission was approached to allow spending a total amount of Rs. 400 million for 2004-2005 on creating facilities, training physicians and support staff and providing ART treatment for 10,000 persons during the year. Half of that would be met from the domestic budget under NACP II and remaining from the technical cooperation component provided by USAID and other donors. The cost of ARV drugs was kept as Rs. 10,000 per patient per year. The initial beneficiaries identified were people living with AIDS who seek treatment in government hospitals, seropositive mothers who participate in the PMTCT programme and children with AIDS younger than 15 years.

We decided to utilise the services of Dr. Bharat Rewari, an experienced physician who was running an ART clinic in RML Hospital, Delhi, to support the ART initiative. Rewari was treating AIDS patients in the RML clinic regularly under the guidance of Dr. Durga Sengupta, a pioneer in management of AIDS cases in Delhi, and had developed a good expertise in ART programming. But it was not until April 2004 that the first patient was provided ART under the national programme, and in the first year only 7000 patients could be covered under ART from 25 centres. That much of lead time was required to carry on the preparatory work, viz establishment of the clinics, training of doctors and nurses, procurement and supply of ARV drugs and diagnostics and expansion of VCTCs. The number of centres was increased to 107 by the end of NACP II. Rewari joined the NACO in January 2005 to lead the ART programme for the next 10 years.

'The programme went through an expansion phase in NACP III. The Global Fund approved grants for free coverage of ART in six high prevalence states in Round IV and later to the entire country in Round VI. 'In 2006, CD 4 testing was made free and dispersible Fixed Dose Combinations (FDCs) of paediatric ARVs were launched. Second line ART was introduced in January 2008, and care of HIV exposed child and Early Infant Diagnosis (EID) launched in 2010. To provide structured training and enhance research, concept of Centers of Excellence (CoEs) was implemented in 2008 and later expanded to paediatric Centers of Excellence PCoEs also. In order to provide services nearer to patient's place of residence, the Link ART Centers (LAC) were conceptualized in May 2008 and upgraded to LAC plus in 2010 to provide pre-ART care as well. The concept of ART plus was devised in October 2010 in order to increase access to second line ART. The supply chain was decentralized in 2012 to SACS for better monitoring of stocks and preventing stock outs. The involvement of community in form of Care Coordinator at all ART centers and GIPA coordinators at SACS went a long way in reducing the stigma and making service more patient friendly'.

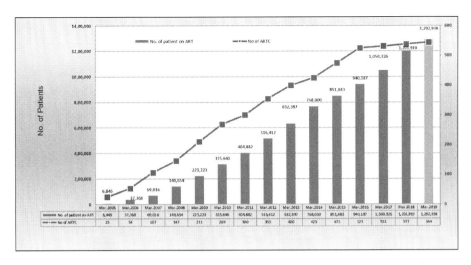

Figure 2: *ART scale-up for PLHIV in India, 2005-2015.*
Source: National AIDS Control Organisation (NACO). Annual Report. Fig. 9.2. Available at:
http://naco.gov.in/sites/default/files/Annual%20Report%202015-16_NACO.pdf

Starting from a modest coverage of about 7000 people, India's ART programme was developed into one of the largest in the world which ultimately covered 1.2 million AIDS patients by 2018. The year-wise cost of ARV drugs got reduced to Rs. 4197 per patient by 2010, which facilitated large-scale expansion of treatment coverage. As the programme expanded the mortality rates started dropping from an all-time high of 230,000 in 2005 to 69,000 in 2017.Only four states, Andhra Pradesh, Telangana, Maharashtra and Karnataka accounted for 53% (37,000) of these deaths.

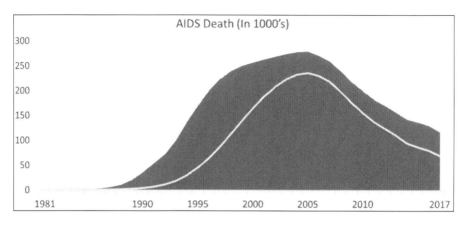

Figure 3: *HIV estimations 2017–National Results (AIDS Deaths).*

In 2014, India completed 10 years of ART programme which was commemorated by NACO with the presence of many of the previous DGs, members of civil society, PLHAs and UNAIDS and other multisectoral donors. I attended the function and shared the enthusiasm with other participants. It was one of the great success stories in disease prevention and control efforts, saving millions of people from disease and death.

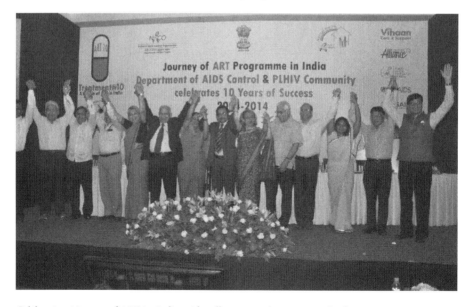

Celebrating 10 years of ART in India with colleagues and community leaders

AVAHAN PROGRAMME

The prevention programme got a boost with Bill and Melinda Gates Foundation (BMGF), showing interest in joining the national efforts. Bill Gates, the Microsoft chief and one of the biggest philanthropists for health sector, visited India in November 2002 and announced a large grant of $200 million (later enhanced to $250 million) from BMGF for containing the HIV epidemic in India and strengthening India's AIDS response. I was heading the Department of Family Welfare in the Ministry and heard that the government was not very receptive to the grant as Bill Gates wanted the money to be spent directly on the programme and not through the government budget. Under NACP II external donors agreed to route their assistance through the NACP budget and the government was not willing to make an exception for Bill Gates. The stalemate continued for some time until Sushma Swaraj joined as the Health Minister in January 2003. For me also, this was one of the first AIDS-related issue I had to handle after taking over as Health Secretary.

The newly appointed India Director of Gates programme, Ashok Alexander, met me to explain the dilemma. He was concerned about the response of the GOI and NACO, which may result in India losing a huge grant entirely meant for prevention of HIV among vulnerable populations. That was my concern too as the NACP II allocations for prevention were not adequate to obtain optimum coverage of targeted populations. I suggested to Alexander that the BMGF should agree to partner with the government to steer the programme in the initial years and obtain consent of all states where they want to work for a fair distribution of project sites between the BMGF and SACS. Health Minister Sushma Swaraj was receptive to the idea of partnership and joint monitoring and agreed to the constitution of a National Steering Committee with me and a BMGF representative cochairing the Committee. The Committee met for the first time and worked out the modalities of implementation. BMGF wanted to work in six states; the southern states of Tamil Nadu, Andhra Pradesh, Karnataka and Maharashtra and the two NE states of Manipur and Nagaland where the epidemic was concentrated.

The next challenge was to make the SACS agree to share the project districts. This was not an easy task as the NACP II was operating in full swing and the SACS were already implementing a large number of prevention programmes for vulnerable populations in all the districts. I wrote to the health secretaries and PD SACS of the six states about BMGF's programme and travelled with Alexander to some of the states namely Tamil Nadu and Andhra Pradesh to work out the modalities. In each of the states the SACS was asked to allocate some of the districts for the BMGF programme for the vulnerable populations. The SACS would continue to do their normative work in the entire state and attend to other programmes such as blood safety, IEC and surveillance in the BMGF districts. Within the next few months the project districts were identified and by December 2004, the BMGF project named 'Avahan' was launched in 83 districts in the six project states.

Avahan had a readymade model of targeted interventions (TIs) for vulnerable communities developed by NACO in 1999 as an important prevention strategy. Avahan improved this model with stronger managerial inputs and closer monitoring and periodic evaluations. Alexander gave strong leadership by travelling extensively in the project districts and interacting with communities and civil society representatives. He and his team had developed a good working relationship with NACO and SACS where the project was in operation. By the time I left the Government in December 2004, Avahan had started actual implementation of interventions, and I was satisfied that the prevention programmes under NACP II got a boost with Avahan complementing governmental efforts in the six project states.

'During the peak implementation phase Avahan provided funding and support to approximately 200 targeted HIV prevention interventions (TIs) across more than 600 towns in 82 districts in six states, covering approximately 200,000 female sex workers (FSW), 80,000 men who have sex with men (MSM) and transgenders, and 20,000 injecting drug users.'[13]

It therefore surprised me that even before the initial 5-year project period came to an end, Avahan was preparing the ground for transfer of the project to NACO. The objective got shifted from complementing national response to demonstration of programmes with coverage and quality and 'graceful transfer' of programmes to NACO without disruption.

This move which was not explicitly stated at the time of launch had surprised everyone. Prevention programmes for HIV have long gestation periods and the results in terms of reduced prevalence would show only after a prolonged period of interventions with the key populations. It would have been proper for Avahan to continue working for a few more years–at least until the MDG Summit of 2015 to produce an impact. But the organisation was in a hurry to close the programme and limit their involvement to provision of technical support only.

The decision to transfer the programme back to NACO did not prove to be a farsighted one. The intervention models followed by NACO and Avahan are qualitatively similar but widely divergent in unit costs and the management of programmes. While NACO was spending about $5 per beneficiary as overhead costs, Avahan spent $18 per beneficiary. NACO's interventions were much larger than Avahan's and it would be difficult for NACO to rework its unit costs to match that of Avahan. NACO was finding it difficult to absorb the transferred programmes and Avahan ultimately agreed to a phased transfer. Avahan was fortunate that the GOI agreed to take over the responsibility for management and financing the large project, despite serious doubts and misgivings about the timing and process of transition. A 2009 Memorandum of Cooperation between the NACO and the BMGF, which was built on an earlier 2006 Memorandum of Understanding (MOU) set out clear agreements regarding the transition process, with 10% of TIs to be transferred to government by April 2009, a further 20% by April 2011, and the remaining 70% by April 2012.

This was essentially a political decision involving high level of commitment of resources and personnel and couldn't be assured despite the 2009 MOU. An evaluation done by John Hopkins University, United States and NACO in 2015 showed that 'transitioning a donor-run program into a government health system was likely to create adaptations in the government system as well as compel adaptation in the program itself. This begs the question as to which adaptations were an acceptable, or even necessary part of transition, and which were likely to damage the long-run sustainability of program outcomes. While TI program managers had positive impressions of program transition, the views of community members were much less so and the community mobilization component of the program suffered most as a consequence of transition'.[14]

In my editorial in STI of *British Medical Journal*, I had suggested that 'instead of "re nationalizing" a well run programme, Avahan should have developed a new public private partnership model for taking over their programmes and running with joint NACO/Avahan partnership. The managerial expertise that Alexander and his colleagues brought to Avahan could have been better utilized to develop such a model as a best practice in the entire Asia Pacific region. As a matter of fact the Commission on AIDS in Asia in its report had advocated for such a model for implementing prevention programmes for key populations for maximum effectiveness'.[15]

In terms of impact, there were two sets of evaluation studies done to estimate the number of infections averted through the Avahan interventions. One study done by the Seattle-based Institute of Health Matrices and Evaluation (IHME) and PHFI India in 2011 put the number of infections averted as 100,000 in a period of 5 years (2003-2008).[16]

The second study done by the Imperial College of London in 2013, put the number as 200,000 in the first 4 years which could go up to 600,000 in 10 years.[17]

These widely varying figures only show how difficult it was to arrive at an accurate estimate of averted infections without a baseline survey which Avahan did not conduct. Avahan was also not working in isolation in the project districts. The footprint of the large national programme (NACP II&III) was present in the Avahan districts too. The enabling sociopolitical environment, the willingness of the state governments to accommodate and work with an external agency and the large IEC and mass awareness campaigns such as the FHAC all had a contribution in reduction of new infections in the project districts. While working in partnership with such a large national programme it would be difficult to attribute impact results to one subset of interventions. The evaluations suffered from this deficiency and did not rightly produce the desired result.

But during its implementation Avahan could generate great amount of visibility for itself and also for the third phase of national programme (NACP III) in the global context. National and foreign media, international funding agencies and UNAIDS were all very appreciative of the focused approach on prevention and close association with the vulnerable and marginalised populations. Avahan's relations with the national programme were also very constructive and friendly.

Contrary to this general impression, Avahan faced criticism for poor referrals of HIV-positive persons from their programmes to the ART centres for treatment. This had deprived ART services to large number of PLHAs among the high-risk populations affecting their right to treatment and good health. Avahan was also not promoting condoms aggressively in their programmes at a time when condoms were the only prevention tool available for protection from HIV.

Avahan has now been completely phased out except for a small component of technical support to NACO to attend to transitional issues. Opinions might be divided on the lasting impact of Avahan on the national programme. But it can't be denied that at a crucial phase of national programme, Avahan had added a strong external component to the prevention programme during implementation of NACP III.

CHANGE OF GUARD IN MINISTRY OF HEALTH

In May 2004, the country went through the next round of parliamentary elections and against all expectations the NDA government led by an able PM Atal Behari Vajpayee lost the elections. A new political formation, the United Progressive Alliance (UPA) led by the Congress party formed the government with Dr. Manmohan Singh as the PM. We were eagerly awaiting the appointment of the Health Minister and expected a senior political functionary from the Congress party to assume the important health portfolio. But under the coalition arrangements, it had gone to a regional political outfit from Tamil Nadu called Pattali Makkal Katchi (PMK) and Dr. Ambumani Ramadoss, a young medical doctor from the party was appointed as the Health Minister with Cabinet rank. Interestingly PMK was a member of the earlier coalition under NDA and two of their functionaries worked as health ministers in the Vajpayee government also. Ramadoss was the third health minister from the regional party, but under a different political formation.

I was left with a tenure of another 6 months before retirement and had to go through the process of adjusting to the new dispensation the third time as a Secretary to the GOI within a span of 3 years. But Minister Ramadoss put me at ease by reposing confidence in me and asking me to keep him regularly updated on the priorities and challenges of a large ministry like health. He was also sufficiently aware of the Ministry's work through his former PMK colleagues who were health ministers. We shared a cordial working relationship until my retirement in December 2004.

I decided to utilise the short period I had to prioritise my work and not spent too much time on regulatory matters. Leadership in NACO was a matter of priority as the incumbent, Meenakshi Dutta Ghosh, was transferred to the Planning Commission. The government decided to appoint S.Y. Quraishi as the new Director of NACO. I was happy to see the leadership passing on to Quraishi who was well known in government circles as an able administrator. His work as DG Doordarshan, the public TV broadcaster, was widely recognised and appreciated. I advised him to bring in Bharat Rewari as the head of the ART programme in NACO as the treatment programme was set for a massive scale-up.

The second phase of NACP II was to end by July 2004. But the government and the World Bank along with other external donors decided to extend the programme for a further period of 18 months until March 2006, as the full complement of committed funds could not be utilised during the 5-year period. 'Re-allocation of funds between categories occurred twice during the project period - once in August 2004 and again in February 2006. Both these actions were largely due to expenditure and disbursement lags, caused by (i) low allocations to the project from the Planning Commission; (ii) capacity constraints at state level in absorbing funds made available by NACO; and (iii) availability of large amounts of additional funding from other donor agencies like the Global Fund'.[18]

OUTCOMES OF NACP II

By the time it ended in 2006 there was an overall sense of achievement as the NACP II had achieved results which could not be anticipated when it was launched in 1999. The concern was that India would end up with as large as 20 million infections if the project fails to deliver. The overall objective for keeping the prevalence under check was to see that the levels are kept within 5% in high prevalence states of Andhra Pradesh, Tamil Nadu, Karnataka, Maharashtra, Manipur and Nagaland and 3% in the rest of India. The Implementation Completion Report (ICR) of the World Bank stated that the overall prevalence has been kept at 0.91% much below the modest targets. This was against an assumed prevalence rate of 0.8% when the project started. There were of course interstate differentials. 'NACO had determined that the epidemic had declined since 1999 in 13 states, remained constant in nine states, and increased in 13 states. The states that performed well were among those with high HIV prevalence, and the reduction in the rate of growth of HIV infection in those states had influenced the overall national trends'. [18] It showed that the march of the AIDS epidemic was virtually halted in India within a period of 7 years. This was no mean achievement for a country with 1.2 billion population with large diversities. In many ways NACP II was responsible in checking a runaway AIDS epidemic in India and laying the foundation for a more organised and expanded response in later years.

It was only later while working in UNAIDS I realised that by innovating from scratch without any previous knowledge or guidance we were able to mount one of the most comprehensive AIDS responses in India. All the important components which were crucial to an effective response found a place in NACP II. The World Bank and other donors acknowledged that a high sense of political commitment, administrative leadership and a contingent of trained and skilled staff were all present in states that had excelled in performance. The central role of surveillance and strategic information, from generation to dissemination and effective programmatic use were all highlighted in the completion report of the World Bank. Most important of all, the strong and effective role played by NGOs and CBOs and the healthy relationship between them and NACO that had evolved and nurtured was the most unique feature of NACP II, not experienced before in any public health programme in India. The TI model which was developed from scratch to provide prevention and care and support services to vulnerable populations was the single most important contributory factor to the success of prevention efforts and for keeping the prevalence levels below 1% in the general population. The number of TIs which were 157 at the start of the project was scaled-up to more than a thousand by 2006. Similarly the number of counselling and testing centres was scale-up from 62 to 1114 during the project period.

The World Bank as the major funding agency applauded the impressive results in its ICR of NACP II. The report says, 'NACO was able to establish its credibility as an entity capable of managing a large program, attracting and managing a large amount of support from a range of donors. NACO was able to expand its program to include many new elements (for example ART and PPTCT) which had not been envisaged under NACP II, initiate new programs namely the sentinel surveillance and BSS to enhance the understanding of the epidemic, and keep the program largely on course. During NACP II it expanded from a fairly modest program focused on blood safety to one of the largest HIV prevention programs in the world'.

The cumulative impact of all these efforts prevented India from becoming a hyper epidemic country as many experts within India and outside predicted. A later study done by the World Bank showed that because of the efforts of successive phases of NACP, 3 million new infections were averted in India by from 1995 till 2015.[19]

Despite all its success it was still an unfinished work that needed to be sustained and further expanded in the next phase of the response. The performance of all the states had not been uniform. States such as Bihar, Madhya Pradesh, Rajasthan and the northeastern states of Manipur and Nagaland did not effectively strengthen the programme management capacity in the SACS. Frequent transfers of programme managers and positioning of junior and inexperienced managers in SACS contributed to slowing down of implementation and non-utilisation of programme funds during later years. The time lag between release of funds by NACO and utilisation at the state level increased as the project rolled on into the last 2 to 3 years. Allocations to NACO also did not keep pace with the amount provided in the original PIP.

It was therefore time to start working on the continuation of the programme into the next phase with greater emphasis on strengthening the capacity at the state level and below for a long and sustained response. The success of NACP II prompted the World Bank to renew their commitment with a larger assistance for the third phase and other donors also followed. The Global Fund which was a strong player in the aid scenario by that time was also keen to support India's large ART programme. Quraishi and I initiated the process of project preparation by constituting a project formulation team to start working on the third phase of the programme. Sadhana Rout, the joint director in charge of IEC and TIs in NACO was brought into the project formulation team to strengthen the civil society component.

Quraishi had also changed the designation of the Project Director of NACO to Director General (DG) to raise the profile of the organisation internationally and within the GOI. I was confident that he would provide able leadership to the national efforts in the years to come.

During the last few months of my stay in the Ministry of Health I focused my attention on the larger public health scenario in the country and building the capacity of institutions engaged in public health programmes.

PUBLIC HEALTH FOUNDATION OF INDIA

A striking feature of India's health scenario was the absence of a critical mass of public health professionals who could inform policy and planning at the national and state levels. The health care system both in public and private sector contained a number of highly qualified clinicians but their involvement and contribution to policy planning was minimal. During my interaction with health professionals from developed countries especially United States, I could feel their deep sense of involvement in policy research and education. Drawn from various branches of medical and nonmedical backgrounds they were in the forefront in formulating health policies and programmes in their own countries and at global level. In comparison, India had very limited pool of talent in public health. The Preventive and Social Medicine (PSM) branch of graduate medical schools was the least preferred option for a medical graduate. Barring one or two, there were no dedicated schools for public health education at that time. With expansion of public health programmes for control of communicable diseases and reproductive health programmes the demand for qualified public health professionals grew enormously. Clinicians with no public health education or training were posted as programme officials at district, state and even national levels to manage large national health programmes. They belonged to the central or state health service cadres and were routinely posted without any relation with their academic qualification or experience. Except the state of Tamil Nadu there were no dedicated cadres of public health professionals in any state at that time. Even in the GOI the Directorate General of Health Services (DGHS) had a small public health sub-cadre inadequate to provide required number of professionals for the top management jobs in the Ministry of Health.

For the first time, the National Health Policy 2002 had pointed to the need to encourage public health education and research. The policy gave opportunity to the nonmedical technical personnel with required qualification to be a part of public health sector. There was some opposition from medical professionals for throwing open the public health career opportunity to nonmedical professionals, but the government decided to go ahead with this important policy change.

My thoughts on this issue got a boost with a chance meeting with Dr. Y. Venugopal Reddy, a senior civil servant who was just appointed as the Governor of Reserve Bank of India, the equivalent of the Federal Reserve in United States. Venugopal Reddy invited me and Dr. Srinath Reddy, the Head of the Cardiology Department in AIIMS, Delhi, for a discussion on public health issues in India and the need to promote public health education and research by creating an autonomous institution outside the control of the government. He was confident that such an initiative could invite private sector funding and be financially viable.

A similar meeting with Rajat Gupta, former chief executive officer (CEO) of McKinseys, also strengthened my views on institution building for public health in India. Rajat Gupta was a member of the Board of the Global Fund for AIDS, TB and Malaria (GFATM) representing private sector. In course of a meeting we had to discuss GFATM and AIDS matters, Rajat Gupta brought up the issue of establishment of an autonomous institution for public health in India. Gupta was of course keen that government should be involved as a partner as the largest market for public health personnel lies in government institutions. Both these meetings encouraged me to pursue the idea of an autonomous public health institution as a new policy initiative.

Time was running out as I had only a few more months left in the Ministry of Health before my retirement. I raised the issue with the new Health Minister Ramadoss and he was equally enthusiastic. His response encouraged me to convene a national consultation for promoting public health in India in September 2004. The Minister attended the consultation and supported the initiative. Representatives from the Association of Schools Public Health (ASPH) in United States and several public health professionals from India and abroad attended the consultation. There was all round enthusiasm and support for starting such an autonomous institution for public health in India.

Follow-up was also quick. Rajat Gupta promised support from McKinseys on a pro bono basis to work out the management model of such an institutional mechanism and placed a team of professionals led by Gautam Kumra to work with us. Srinath Reddy and I spent 2 full days with the McKinseys team to evolve the institutional mechanism. After intense consultations a model institutional structure was evolved with strong presence of both public and private sectors but outside the control of government. A public private partnership (PPP) model was worked out consisting of members from senior levels in Ministry of Health, PMO, Planning Commission and Ministry of Science and Technology as ex officio members. Other members should be from public health professionals, civil society and private sector. The Chair should be from outside the Government and a senior health care professional should head the organisation as the CEO. The organisation would be registered as a society under the Society Registration Act 1860. With a basic framework emerging from the discussions, Srinath and Gautam Kumra assumed responsibility to pursue the proposal in the Ministry of Health after my retirement.

FRAMEWORK CONVENTION ON TOBACCO CONTROL (FCTC)

My 7 years' tenure in Ministry of Health as Additional Secretary and PD NACO and later as Secretary Health and Family Welfare was a great opportunity to participate and pursue a number of global initiatives for disease control. Prominent were the TB and malaria control programmes which had a major funding from the World Bank. But the most exciting work of those years was the emergence of the Framework Convention on Tobacco Control (FCTC) from a major initiative taken by WHO under the leadership of DG Gro Harlem Bruntland. She established the Tobacco-Free Initiative in WHO and in May 1999, the World Health Assembly paved the way to multilateral negotiations on establishing a FCTC. A Technical Working Group (TWG) and an intergovernmental negotiating body were established to draft and negotiate the Convention and related protocols. The negotiating body met for the first time in October 2000, and elected Ambassador Celso Amorim from Brazil as the Chair. India was one of the Vice Chairs along with five other countries including the United States. The negotiating body met six times between October 2000 and March 2003. I got the opportunity to lead the Indian delegation to the negotiations with Srinath Reddy and Srinivas Tata, the Director, looking after tobacco issues in the ministry. We as a delegation played an important role in advocating for strong anti-tobacco measures including a total ban on tobacco advertising, public smoking and providing health messages on cigarettes, *bidis* and chewing tobacco products. We as a team conducted successful regional consultations among WHO SEARO countries and brought unanimity in approach among all the 11 SEARO nations on tobacco control issues in the negotiating body.

On May 21, 2003, the World Health Assembly finally adopted the landmark FCTC and opened it for signing and ratification by member countries. It was the first global convention steered by WHO and was a crowning achievement for its DG Gro Harlem Bruntland who provided excellent leadership to the efforts of countries to regulate tobacco use.

India was one of the first nations to sign the Convention in 2004. But our tobacco control efforts even predated the signing of the convention. We initiated legislative action for tobacco control in 2003 with the enactment of the Cigarettes and Other Tobacco Products (Prohibition of Advertisement and Regulation of Trade and Commerce, Production, Supply and Distribution) Act, 2003 (COTPA) which contained many measures to discourage use of tobacco and tobacco products.

Successive health ministers, Sushma Swaraj and Ambumani Ramadoss, provided strong leadership in getting the national legislation enacted and brought into force. My last act in the ministry was the release of a well-researched Ministry publication 'Tobacco Use in India' which was compiled in record time by Dipankar Gupta and Srinath Reddy to coincide with my departure from the ministry.

Many of these initiatives needed strong follow-up. But that was for someone else to take care of as I retired from the government as the Health Secretary on 30 November 2004, at the age of 60 years. It was a long journey from 1967 when I joined the IAS at the age of 22 as a young aspiring member with a master's degree in Nuclear Physics. The journey took me from the remote rural areas of West Bengal to the Writers Building, the historic secretariat of West Bengal Government, to the Indian capital Delhi for the last lap of 7 years in the GOI, in the Ministry of Health and Family Welfare.

My family joined me in commemorating this journey by arranging my *Shasti Poorthi* in Vijayawada, Andhra Pradesh, an Indian custom for celebrating completion of a 60-year cycle in Indian calendar.

REFERENCES

1. An excerpt from Chief Minister Chandrababu Naidu's speech. Available at: http://www.policyproject.com/pubs/generalreport/ANE_ActNow.pdf

2. Jana S, Basu I, Rotheram-Borus MJ, Newman PA. The Sonagachi Project: a sustainable community intervention program. *AIDS Educ Prev* 2004 Oct;16(5):405-14. doi: 10.1521/aeap.16.5.405.48734

3. United Nations Office on Drugs and Crime, Regional Office for South Asia. Women who use drugs in Northeast India. 2015. Available at: https://www.unodc.org/documents/southasia/publications/research-studies/FINAL_REPORT.pdf

4. Sarkar S, Das N, Panda S, Naik TN, Sarkar K, Singh BC, et al. Rapid spread of HIV among injecting drug users in north-eastern states of India. *Bull Narc.* 1993;45(1):91-105.

5. Report submitted by NACO for World Bank completion mission for NACP II. March 2006, Available at: http://naco.gov.in/sites/default/files/The%20 World%20Bank%20Appraisal%20of%20NACP%20III.pdf

6. "Civilities, What does the acronym LGBTQ stand for?". Washington Post. Retrieved February 19, 2018.

7. The History and Activism of the LGBTQ Community in India Utsa Sarmin. The Wire 10 September 2018. Available at: https://www.telesurenglish. net/analysis/The-History-and-Activism-of-LGBTQ-Community-in-India-20180909-0009.html

8. Lawyers Collective. Legal officer for the HIV/AIDS Unit. May 23, 2018. Available at: https://lawyerscollective.org/2018/05/23/legal-officer-for-the-hivaids-unit/

9. Durban Declaration. *Nature.* 406 (6791);15-16:2000. doi:10.1038/35017662. PMID 10894520.

10. UN Security Council Resolution 1308 (2000) on the Responsibility of the Security Council in the Maintenance of International Peace and Security: HIV/AIDS and International Peace-keeping Operations. 2000.

11. Centre for Reproductive Rights. UNGASS on HIV/AIDS: Women's Empowerment Embraced, Reproductive Rights Slighted. 2001. Available at: http://reproductiverights.org/sites/default/files/documents/pub_bp_ UNGASS.pdf

12. Human Rights Watch-Ignorance only -HIV/AIDS Human Rights and federally funded abstinence only programmes in United States-Texas: a case study. 2002;14:no 5G.

13. Verma R, Shekhar A, Khobragade S, Adhikary R, George B, Ramesh BM, et al. Scale-up and coverage of Avahan: a large-scale HIV-prevention programme among female sex workers and men who have sex with men in four Indian states. *Sex Transm Infect.* 2010;86:i76-82. doi: 10.1136/sti.2009.039115 PMID: 20167737.

14. Bennett S, Singh S, Rodriguez D, Ozawa S, Singh K, Chhabra V, et al. Transitioning a large scale HIV/AIDS prevention program to local stakeholders: findings from the Avahan transition evaluation. *PLOS ONE.* September 1, 2015. Available at: https://doi.org/10.1371/journal. pone.0136177

15. Rao JVRP. Avahan: the transition to a publicly funded programme as a next stage. *Sex Transm Infect.* 2010 Feb;86:i7-8. doi: 10.1136/sti.2009.039297.

16. Gakidou E, Murray CJL, Dandona L. HIV/AIDS prevention initiative averts 100,000 infections in India. IHME October 11, 2011. Available at: http://www.healthdata.org/news-release/hivaids-prevention-initiative-averts-100000-infections-india

17. Wong S. Avahan AIDS initiative may have prevented 600,000 HIV infections in India. Imperial College of London. September 30, 2013. Available at: https://www.imperial.ac.uk/news/130953/avahan-aids-initiative-have-prevented-600000/

18. World Bank Report on Credit to India for NACP II. Implementation completion and results report. September 20, 2006. South Asia Human Development Sector. World Bank Office: New Delhi. Available at: https://www.scribd.com/document/77769497/The-World-Bank-Report-on-Credit-to-India-for-NACP-II

19. A World Bank Policy Research Report. Confronting AIDS: Public priorities in a global epidemic. The World Bank. Washington, D.C. 1997. Available at: http://documents1.worldbank.org/curated/en/241011468155717656/pdf/multi0page.pdf

CHAPTER 3

STIMULATING THE REGIONAL RESPONSE IN ASIA PACIFIC

In June 2004, I travelled to Geneva to attend the board meeting of Global Fund on AIDS, Tuberculosis and Malaria (GFATM). India was representing the South East Asia Regional Office (SEARO) constituency in the Fund Board and it was my first meeting with the board as Secretary Health in Government of India. I met Peter Piot and during a private conversation he informed me about his plans to decentralise the governance structure in Joint United Nations Programme on HIV/AIDS (UNAIDS) and delegate more authority to countries and regions to provide them with a larger share of technical resources and reduce staff strength in Geneva. He was planning to establish regional support teams in different regions, two for Africa, one each for Asia Pacific, Latin America, Eastern Europe and Central Asia and for the Caribbean region. He wanted to start the Asia Pacific regional support team (RST) in Bangkok by merging the two small technical support units in Delhi and Bangkok into one. He wanted me to join UNAIDS as the regional director in Bangkok.

Peter and I had shared a warm and friendly relationship all these years since we met in 1997, but I had never anticipated that I would get an offer to work in his organisation. I was a rank outsider to the UN system and had never worked outside of India. Most important, I still had 6 months of tenure left in the government at the senior position of Union Health Secretary. At a time when I should be giving my best efforts to the Government of India I did not want to leave the job midway for a UN assignment. But Peter had answers to all my doubts. He was keen in getting me as I was sufficiently familiar with UNAIDS and developed good understanding of its work at country and headquarters level. It should not be difficult to get to know the work at regional level. He was prepared to keep the position vacant until my retirement in November 2004.

It was such a sudden development that it took me some time to evaluate the options. My first priority was to work in India in health sector-related programmes. The Public Health Foundation of India (PHFI) and Tobacco Control were great initiatives, but I could not spot a role where I could fit in. The PHFI was still on the drawing board and might take another year to get off the ground whereas the Tobacco initiative was entirely a government-controlled system. I was greatly encouraged by friends in UNAIDS to take up the assignment as it would provide an opportunity to put my experience in India's national programme to good use in other countries in the region. After much thought I decided to take the plunge and informed Peter that I would be joining the assignment within a month's time after my retirement on 30 November 2004.

After completing all post-retirement formalities, I travelled to Bangkok and took charge of the RST of UNAIDS on 20 December 2004. The office located on the 9th floor of UN building on Rajadamnern Avenue, still housed the former intercountry team (ICT) with a small contingent of technical staff who were internationals and five or six Thai nationals as supporting staff. With the amalgamation of Delhi office, some of the international staff from Delhi were repositioned to Bangkok. More technical staff was expected to join in the next couple of months.

UNAIDS COSPONSOR RELATIONS

I was familiar with UNAIDS through my work with Geneva and the country office in India, but did not have intimate knowledge of its internal working processes. I had no familiarity with the dynamics of the relation of the secretariat as UNAIDS was known with the cosponsor

UN organisations which increased in number to 10 from the 6 original cosponsors mentioned in the Economic and Social Council (ECOSOC) resolution of 1994. The council in its resolution had declared that the joint programme would 'strengthen the capacity of the United Nations system to monitor trends and ensure that appropriate and effective policies and strategies are implemented at the country level, strengthen the capacity of national Governments to develop comprehensive national strategies and implement effective HIV/AIDS activities at the country level, promote broad-based political and social mobilization to prevent and respond to HIV/AIDS within countries and advocate greater political commitment in responding to the epidemic at the global and country levels, including the mobilization and allocation of adequate resources for HIV/AIDS-related activities.'[1]

The relation between the cosponsors and the programme was a two-way process as envisaged by ECOSOC. The resolution specifies that 'the co-sponsors will share responsibility for the development of the programme, contribute equally to its strategic direction and receive from it, policy and technical guidance relating to the implementation of their HIV/AIDS activities'. The programme director would work under the overall guidance of a Programme Coordinating Board (PCB) which was established by another ECOSOC resolution 1995/223 with 22 member countries and 6 members of the cosponsors who work together as a Committee of Cosponsoring Organisations (CCOs). Nongovernment organisations' (NGOs) participation was limited to five members, three from the developing countries and two from the developed countries. Eligibility criteria for selection of NGOs were also specified in the resolution.

At the country level it was recognised that the ultimate responsibility for responding to the epidemic lies with the national governments and the joint programme will provide coordinated support through a Theme Group (TG) of all the cosponsors. To coordinate the activities of the cosponsors a staff member will be recruited who will assist the TG Chair to manage the coordinated programme in support of country's requirements. The position of Country Programme Advisor (CPA) was created progressively in most of the countries.

But within the closed doors of the UN system, a bitter struggle was being fought by the fledgling secretariat with World Health Organization (WHO) which did not take kindly to the Global Programme on AIDS (GPA) being taken out of their jurisdiction. Other cosponsor agencies also did not want a strong secretariat to take control of the joint programme. The secretariat had struggled hard during the initial years to stabilise the relationship between the cosponsors and secretariat. But Peter's committed leadership and the support and confidence he enjoyed with Kofi Annan, the new UN Secretary-General (SG), enabled him to steer the programme through rough weather. The United Nations General Assembly Special Session (UNGASS) 2001 and the Security Council resolutions lifted the AIDS agenda to the top of political discourse. GFATM and the President's Emergency Plan for AIDS Relief (PEPFAR) of US government increased the resource commitment to billions from the meagre $500 million that could be mustered for global AIDS response until 2000. All along this journey, the strong message given was that AIDS was an exceptional disease and needed an exceptional response. A biomedical approach will not produce results. The key to success will be the close involvement of communities of affected populations and people living with HIV not as beneficiaries but partners in governance. Peter pursued the concept of AIDS exceptionalism relentlessly for the next 10 years with astonishing drive and commitment.

The organisation also expanded with emphasis on strong country-level presence in problem countries. The position of CPA was upgraded as UNAIDS country coordinator (UCC) and later as UNAIDS Country Director (UCD), giving it equal status with the heads of other UN agencies at country level. Areas such as strategic information, monitoring and evaluation, prevention and involvement of communities were all brought to prominence in the secretariat functioning. Peter was successful in scouting for good talent across the globe and inducted personnel from diverse fields of technical expertise at senior levels in the secretariat. Purnima Mane, Rob Moodie, Jim Sherry, Bernhard Schwartländer, Paul De Lay, Olavi Elo, Karen Stanecki, Werasit Sittitrai and Michel Sidibe were all well-known experts in their fields and constituted the brains trust of UNAIDS secretariat. Michel was looking after country- and regional-level programming as Director of Country Programmes when I assumed charge as Director RST. The headquarters office which was initially functioning from a small annex building adjoining the WHO headquarters got its own office opposite to the WHO building in October 2006.

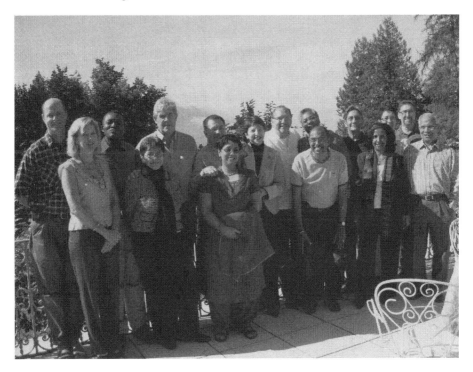

Senior Management Team of UNAIDS with Peter

DECENTRALISATION OF MANAGMENT IN UNAIDS

Peter and Michel were already working on upgrading the intercountry units as full-fledged regional offices in the six regions of Eastern and Southern Africa (ESA), Asia and Pacific (AP), Western and Central Africa (WCA), Eastern Europe and Central Asia (EECA), Latin America and Caribbean (LAC) and Middle East and Northern Africa (MENA). The cosponsors were not entirely happy with opening of full-fledged regional outfits by the secretariat but this sensitive issue was not openly discussed. Peter found a solution by calling them regional support teams to provide technical support to the countries in areas such as strategic information, monitoring and evaluation, political advocacy, resource assessment and community mobilisation. The oversight function of the UNAIDS country offices was later given to the RSTs as a part of the decentralisation process.

By the time I joined as RST Director, the teams in ESA and WCA were already functioning with Mark Stirling who was brought from UNICEF New York office and Meskerem Bekele Grunitzy a tropical diseases researcher from Ethiopia respectively as Directors. The teams in Caribbean and Latin America which initially functioned as separate units were later merged into one and Cesar Nunez, former Director of National AIDS Programme in Honduras, was appointed as Director. Oussama Tawil, already working as team leader in Middle East and North Africa (MENA) inter-country team was appointed as Director for MENA region. It was proving difficult to choose a director for the Moscow-based RST for EECA as UNAIDS did not have many Russian knowing staff on its rolls. Finally, Bertil Lindblad from the UNAIDS office in New York, was posted as the director.

My joining the office on 20 December was immediately followed by a tumultuous event, the Indonesian Tsunami on 25 December 2004. I was staying on the 11th floor of a hotel in central Bangkok and suddenly saw the ceiling fan in the room swaying wildly and the wooden cupboards rattling. There was an earthquake alert and we all were asked to go downstairs. We waited on the footpath outside the hotel for about 30 minutes and returned to the rooms when everything became quiet. By the evening we saw on the TV the devastating impact of the tsunami on Aceh in Indonesia, Phuket and other parts of Thailand. As the tragedy unfolded in the next few days we could see the impact of the tsunami spreading up to the South Indian coast and beyond. The series of tsunamis killed more than 228,000 people and left more than 2 million people homeless. The UN agencies joined the efforts of affected countries with a colossal $6.25 billion donated to a central UN relief fund assisting 14 countries affected by the disaster. The aid response to the tsunami was quite unprecedented. Office for the Coordination of Humanitarian Affairs (OCHA), United Nations Development Programme (UNDP), WHO and United Nations International Children's Emergency Fund (UNICEF) joined the unprecedented relief and rehabilitation efforts at country and regional level. The UNAIDS secretariat did not have a direct role in relief operations, but I used to regularly attend UN coordinating meetings and follow the relief efforts initiated by the various agencies. I designated Taona Nana Kuo, a temporary technical advisor in the RST as the focal point for disaster relief and rehabilitation for Asia Tsunami victims. In our own small way, we tried to provide post-exposure prophylaxis (PEP) kits for the UN personnel working in Tsunami devastated countries to protect them from HIV infection by accidental needle stick injuries.

Meanwhile UNAIDS started pursuing the decentralisation agenda earnestly with strong push coming from Peter. The regional directors (RDs) were asked to join a series of senior management meetings in January 2005, where the policy behind decentralisation was explained in detail. The reorganisation was sought to be carried out in an overall framework of an integrated UNAIDS from country to headquarters. The key results and the value added by the RSTs would be rated as more important than the functions they were going to perform. There was a definite shift from a technical assistance framework to an overall programmatic support to the UNAIDS country directors and through them to the country programmes. Better interaction with regional and intergovernmental bodies would be another area of priority for the RSTs.

I wanted that our work in RST should be closely aligned to the country requirements and this would be possible only when the regional programme advisors in the team (RPAs as they were designated) maintain a close contact with the UCCs and through them with the national programmes. I introduced the system of designating each of the RPA as a country focal point who would be like a one stop shop for all interactions between the RST and the UNAIDS Country Office (UCO). The work plans and travel plans of the RPAs should be aligned to the implementation of the UCO work plan and allied requirements. This also resulted in the reworking of travel plans of some RPAs which initially caused some resentment. But everyone saw the need for reorienting their work to suit the country's needs and acceded to my request to cut down on avoidable travel time.

I then decided to meet the UCCs first in sub-regional groups and then individually. The two meetings I had for South Asia and South East Asia in Delhi and Bangkok were very informative for me as a newcomer to UNAIDS. I had interacted with UCC India, earlier as a Director of the national programme, but in these meetings I could understand the dynamics from UNAIDS' point of view. The most critical issue that struck me was the limitation of the role of a UCC within the overall working of the UN TG consisting of the representatives of all the 10 UNAIDS cosponsors. The perception of many UCCs was that they are accountable to the TG and would act as per the work plan prepared and approved by the TG. Who will then be accountable to the countries, the governments and the civil societies? There were some frank exchange of views on the role of the UCCs vis-a-vis the country programmes and I shared my vision that the UCC should be the first point of call for any requirement of technical support for the national programme. We can't be 'hiding behind the TGs' for all the work that we do at the country level. Cosponsors had their own programmes and it would be too much to expect them to give their full attention to AIDS agenda only. The UCC as the name itself suggested should coordinate the UN support to the country programme and for this sake should be in direct contact with the national programme managers. The level of interaction should also be raised from a managerial and technical level to the political level. Without political support and resource commitment our technical support was not effective. I advised the UCCs that they should try to find new equations with the health ministers and administrative secretaries instead of limiting their interactions to technical managers only and make political advocacy their direct responsibility.

HIV/AIDS SCENARIO IN ASIA PACIFIC

For the first few months I was trying to get familiarised with the diverse nature of AIDS epidemic and responses in different countries in the region. In 2004, HIV/AIDS in Asia Pacific presented a picture of a diverse and growing epidemic. 'An estimated 8.2 million adults and children were living with HIV. About 540 000 people died of AIDS. In countries as diverse as China, India, Indonesia, Malaysia, Nepal, Pakistan, Singapore and Vietnam, national epidemics are concentrated among key vulnerable populations, such as sex workers and their clients, injecting drug users (IDUs), men who have sex with men (MSM), and certain mobile populations. However, the virus could move into the general population unless determined action is taken now' warned the regional report of UNAIDS that came out in mid-2004.[2]

The typical features of the epidemic in the regions were
i.   The epidemic was still concentrated among the key populations vulnerable to HIV, namely sex workers, people who inject drugs and MSM and transgender communities. Clients of sex workers called the bridge populations accounted for a substantial number of new infections.
ii. Prevalence levels were low (< 1%) but even this low prevalence resulted in large number of infected persons in countries namely India and China.
iii. High level of mobility driven by rapid economic advancement in countries was a key driver of new infection rates among young male adults with disposable incomes.

Thailand, and later Cambodia, witnessed early rise of infections followed by other countries such as Indonesia, Vietnam and Myanmar. China was getting impacted by a drug user epidemic largely driven by people who inject drugs. In the Pacific, Papua New Guinea (PNG) was experiencing an alarming rise of HIV, leading to a generalised type of epidemic with 1.7% reported prevalence in general population. The regional report warned that 'More than 50% of adult men report multiple sex partners. The virus is spreading most rapidly in rural areas. The challenges of mounting an effective response to AIDS in Papua New Guinea are daunting—the country has a large number of ethnic groups, multiple languages, and a poorly developed communications infrastructure'.[2] In South Asia, Pakistan and Nepal were reporting increasing number of new infections.

Response of most countries was still inadequate and yet to reach optimum levels for new infections to decrease substantially. Several indicators such as low levels of awareness on HIV/AIDS, suboptimal coverage of prevention interventions, inadequate access to condom promotion campaigns, underdeveloped prevention of mother-to-child transmission of HIV (PMTCT) programmes showed that Asia Pacific countries were lagging behind in responding to a raging epidemic among the most vulnerable populations, young people and migrants. Institutional challenges, like weak political support for AIDS programmes, inadequate financial resources, weak surveillance systems, inadequate involvement of non-health sectors in AIDS programmes and lack of support for Civil Society Organisation (CSO) partners were also hindering a scaled-up response in the region. Thailand undertook a strong initiative that focused on 100% use of condoms by sex workers and their clients, resulting in marked decrease of new infections in these populations. But complacency gave rise to falling resources for prevention programmes in the country. Apart from Thailand, India was the only country which mounted a comprehensive response to the epidemic addressing all risk factors and involving all stakeholders. China which had the second largest prevalence came out of denial mode after the report of UNAIDS 'HIV/AIDS China's Titanic Peril' stirred up a big controversy within the country. There was growing evidence of other countries such as Myanmar, Vietnam, Nepal and Cambodia adopting new strategies for intensifying prevention programmes. But the overall coverage of vulnerable populations with prevention interventions was very low, said the UNAIDS report.[3] But treatment programmes were still beyond the means of most countries in Asia Pacific. Except Thailand, no other country in the region could cover more than 25% of eligible population under antiretroviral therapy (ART) programmes.[4]

But the biggest obstacle to a scaled-up response was the high level of stigma and discrimination against people living with HIV and vulnerable communities in Asia Pacific countries. 'According to a 2003 assessment of national AIDS responses in all regions, Asian countries scored lower on human rights-related issues than in any other category of response component (e.g., prevention, care and impact mitigation). Commitments on paper frequently do not translate into real protection for HIV-positive people'.[2]

UNAIDS identified the challenge as inadequate prevention efforts focused on vulnerable populations by national programmes, resulting in increased incidence levels. In June 2005, UNAIDS prepared a policy position paper on HIV prevention and presented it to the PCB for approval. It was a very comprehensive policy document where the principles of effective prevention programmes and the essential HIV policy and programmatic actions were identified. 'In order to ensure that efforts to intensify HIV prevention can be sustained, UNAIDS will continue to be guided by the centrality of national ownership and the need for a truly multisectoral response.

The paper outlined that in line with its five core functions, UNAIDS will focus on the following areas:

➤ Advocacy on HIV prevention;
➤ Policy development in areas critical for HIV prevention;
➤ Technical support and capacity building for implementation of scaled-up HIV prevention programmes;
➤ Coordination and harmonisation of HIV prevention efforts; and
➤ Tracking, monitoring and evaluation of HIV prevention programmes'.[5]

The status of AIDS epidemic and the regional response reminded me of my time in NACO when I was directly involved in leading the national response some 7 years ago. But my role as RST Director would be different–more as a UN advocate and provider of strategic technical support. But working directly with national programme managers to know their technical and programme requirements and garnering necessary support at country and regional level was essential. Most important was working with senior-level political and administrative leadership to keep priority on AIDS programmes and commit larger resources for prevention and treatment.

THE THREE ONES

During the years following the UNGASS 2001 and creation of GFATM, UNAIDS had come up with a strategy called 'Three Ones', underlying the principles for national level HIV/AIDS coordination, to utilise the resources for maximum impact on global response. The principles were identified through a preparatory process at global and country levels, initiated in cooperation with the World Bank and the GFATM and were further refined in dialogue with other key donor partners.

The three principles applicable to all stakeholders in the country-level HIV/AIDS response were identified as:

➢ **One** agreed HIV/AIDS Action Framework that provides the basis for coordinating the work of all partners.
➢ **One** National AIDS Coordinating Authority, with a broad based multi-sector mandate.
➢ **One** agreed country level Monitoring and Evaluation System.

Simple in its concept and direct in its message, the Three Ones strategy found instant appeal with the country leadership. Many countries started to constitute national AIDS committees as multisectoral entities with government and community participation. An in-house committee within the Health Ministry with the Health Minister as Chair of the Committee was a commonly adopted model, but some countries went ahead raising the profile of the NAC with the prime minister (PM) or minister of coordination chairing the committee. Cambodia, India, Indonesia and Pakistan decided to raise the status of the chair to the PM or a senior cabinet minister in charge of coordination. This move had enabled the UNAIDS leadership to directly engage with political leadership at a very senior level, something which was not achieved earlier.

The second 'one' of a single national strategic plan (NSP) was more challenging. The national plans in number of countries were more like strategy documents without a fully costed implementation plan. There were many impediments in evolving such costed plans. Lack of commitment for sustainable financing of the NSPs and lack of a costing structure for various interventions under the national plans hindered presenting a fully costed NSP for a period of more than 2 years.

A single M&E agency for monitoring the epidemic was still a far cry as many countries still lacked a sound M&E framework for monitoring implementation of all interventions in the national programmes.

But the 'three ones' gave the country and regional offices of UNAIDS a concrete base to work upon and report on outcomes. They also helped to get a better country orientation in formulating their biannual work plans and presenting them to prospective donors for funding such initiatives.

My work in the RST started in the backdrop of these important changes in policy and funding environment which governed the global-level response for the next decade with impressive outcomes.

FIELD VISITS TO PNG AND THE PHILIPPINES

In February 2005, UNAIDS headquarters informed me that Peter would be attending a steering committee meeting of the Asia Pacific Leadership Forum (APLF) in PNG. The forum was established in 2002 following the Asia Pacific Ministerial Meeting in October 2001 in Melbourne, Australia, with an aim to support and strengthen political and civil society leadership at country, sub-regional and regional levels in taking action to reduce the spread and impact of the AIDS epidemic in the region. Members were drawn from different countries in Asia Pacific region representing political leaders, parliamentarians and opinion leaders from civil society. I undertook my first country-level visit to PNG and met many leaders from the region in the meeting, including Nafis Sadik, the Special Envoy of UN SG on AIDS in Asia Pacific and former Executive Director of UNFPA who was a member of the forum. Our association continued until I succeeded her as the Special Envoy some 7 years later in 2012.

Papua New Guinea is the largest of the pacific islands and the most complex in its demography and culture to understand the status of the epidemic and assess the response. Formulating a national response, however, was challenging in a country where 5.1 million people converse with each other in more than 800 languages and are scattered across an area of rugged terrain larger than Japan. Traditional cultures and social controls were breaking down. The growth of a cash economy and urbanisation fostered widespread high-risk behaviour. In PNG sexual activity starts at the age of 15 to 16 for both men and women and an increasing number of both had multiple sex partners, whether inside or outside of marriage. The use of sex to obtain cash, goods or services was also widespread outside the sex industry. High levels of sexually transmitted infections (STIs) showed that condom use was low. A severe economic recession since the 1990s made the problems worse. Soaring poverty caused thousands of rural inhabitants to migrate to urban areas where prostitution and sexual violence had increased. The breakdown of traditional protective customs for women combined with a reluctance to discuss sexual matters complicated prevention and awareness strategies.

Without rapid interventions, the impact of the epidemic would be severe. Papua New Guinea's National Health Plan pointed out that 'if the epidemic is left to run at the present rate of increase, 70% of the hospital beds in the country could be occupied by AIDS patients in 2010'. It also noted that 'at a 10% HIV prevalence rate, tuberculosis will rise 50% to affect 30% of the population'.

Dame Carol Kidu, the Minister for Community Development in PNG said, 'I see people are going to be dying unnecessarily because they don't know how to protect themselves and are held back by the shackles of cultural attitudes. In terms of HIV/AIDS awareness, the government has become irrelevant to many communities because [the communities are] so isolated'.[6]

She took us on some local visits to communities such as the Hetura Youth Development Centre, the Rabiagini Community, a low-income settlement and Pari village, an urban settlement of indigenous Motu language group. The scenes were depressing. Poverty, unemployment and crimes against women compounded the problem of AIDS and the programme was not reaching to the people who needed it most. Most of the work of the government was happening in Port Moresby, the capital city, and very little across the rural hinterland. The main hospital in Port Moresby was flooded with people from different parts of the country seeking antiretroviral (ARV) treatment. The ART drugs were getting procured from generic manufacturers from India but there was no organised procurement mechanism in operation. On the brighter side, PNG had an AIDS legislation, one of the few countries in the region to have a separate HIV/AIDS Act. A National AIDS Council was established and functioning since 1997 with representation from a wide spectrum of stakeholders. A well-articulated National Strategic Plan (NSP) (2004-2008) was in position focusing on seven priority areas of national importance. In the same year a PMTCT programme was introduced covering six hospitals in the country. A very active parliamentary standing committee on AIDS was functioning, led by Dr. Banare Bun, a distinguished parliamentarian of the country. The downside was the poor health care infrastructure in the country which made implementation of the programme extremely difficult. In many remote areas it was virtually nonexistent, leaving it to the local churches to provide palliative health care and support to the infected populations. Nii K Plange, a social scientist from Ghana was the UCC, working against all odds to support the national programme. He was left with a short tenure by the time I joined in Bangkok and moved to Geneva in August 2005.

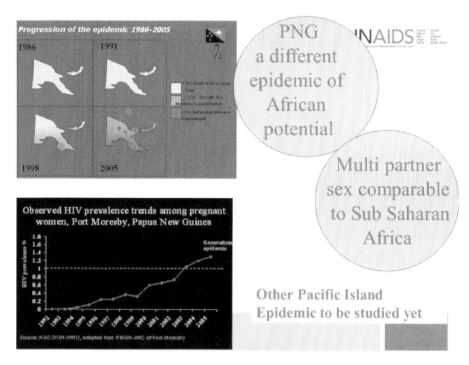

Figure 4: PNG: a different epidemic of African potential–(UNAIDS).

For me it was the first exposure to the remote Pacific Island country and what I saw was a potential African type epidemic not witnessed anywhere in Asia. It could break out into a generalised epidemic with infection levels in general population crossing the 2% mark. Since then PNG always remained as a priority and held my attention more than any other country in the region.

Our next port of call was Manila, where Peter and I met the senior management of Asian Development Bank (ADB) to work out a regional collaboration agreement between UNAIDS and ADB. Peter signed a memorandum of understanding (MOU) between the two organisations and addressed a press conference. We also met President Ramos, former President of Philippines, in a press conference to highlight the importance of leadership in HIV/AIDS. In contrast to PNG, Philippines' AIDS control programme seemed working well with active participation of civil society partners such as Penoy Plus. We met the House Special Committee on millennium development goals (MDGs) to draw their attention to the problem of HIV/AIDS. The partnership with ADB flourished in later years and resulted in establishment of a unique facility–the AIDS Data Hub for Asia Pacific in collaboration with UNICEF Asia regional office.

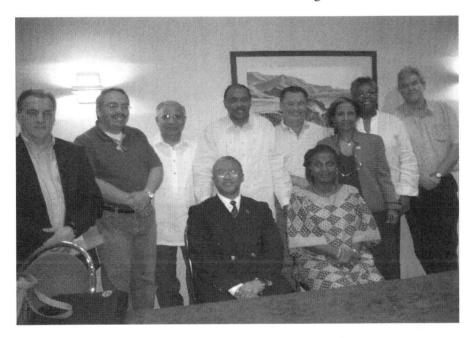

With Michel (fourth from left–standing) and RST Directors at Johannesburg meeting

As I was preparing to return to Bangkok, I got a message about a Programme Planning workshop, Michel called with all the RDs in Johannesburg, South Africa, on 24 and 25 February 2005. I had no time to go back to Bangkok and plan my visit from there. My office connected me from Singapore to Johannesburg on a nonstop 11-hour flight across the Indian Ocean. It was the longest air travel I undertook until then and left me totally exhausted by the time I reached Johannesburg on 24 February. But the meeting I had with fellow RST Directors, many of whom I met for the first time, energised me. We had a stimulating discussion on the role of the RSTs and the delegation of authority needed for their effective functioning. Michel as Director of country and regional support division (CRD) provided able leadership to this group of six RST Directors, from Asia Pacific to Latin

America. We impressed upon him the need to provide adequate financial and administrative powers to the RST Directors if they had to effectively supervise the work at country and regional levels. The RST Directors were later included in the Senior Management Team (SMT) of UNAIDS and contributed substantially to policy development and programme decentralisation. The decisions taken in Johannesburg meeting were pathbreaking and led to effective decentralisation of UNAIDS to country and regional levels.

ICAAP KOBE 2005

An important follow-up from the PNG visit was the revival of the International Conferences on AIDS in Asia Pacific (ICAAP). The ICAAPs were held since 1983 every alternative year and provided civil society space to communities to deliberate on issues connected with AIDS response in the region. They provided an excellent platform for the communities to make their voice heard and to strengthen their networks. After the 2001 Melbourne Conference, Kobe in Japan was chosen for the 2003 meet. The Kobe earthquake devastated the city and the conference was postponed. Not until 2005 could the initiative be revived. Marina Mahathir, chair of the Malaysian AIDS Foundation, and I were asked to visit Kobe and talk to the local organisers to review the preparations for the 2005 ICAAP. We travelled to Kobe and met Masayoshi Tarui and Masahiro Kihara, the cochairs of the local organising committee. The civil society partners and research community in Japan were quite enthusiastic about holding the ICAAP, but their enthusiasm was not matched equally by the government. Marina and I pledged full support from UNAIDS for organising the conference and supporting participation of delegates. We recruited a local consultant to provide full-time support to the local organising committee and to maintain close contact with the RST. Events moved fast and we could organise the 10th ICAAP in July 2005 in Kobe, my first conference as RST Director and a co-organiser.

Peter Piot attended the conference as promised and spoke at the opening ceremony. He encouraged me to present a regional picture on the epidemic and the response pointing out the inadequacies in a frank and forthright manner. I thought this was my best opportunity to present a regional snapshot of the epidemic and the response of Asia Pacific countries which was lagging behind on many fronts. I was the first plenary speaker and made a forthright and provocative presentation supported by country-level data. I highlighted the challenge of poor coverage of key populations with focused prevention and ART programmes and rising resource gap for an effective response (shown in slides). I concluded by calling AIDS in Asia a 'Silent Tsunami' and that the region will miss a great opportunity if timely action was not taken. The word 'tsunami' struck a chord with the Japanese media who were silent until then. I was immediately confronted by some reporters to explain why I called the epidemic a tsunami. Next day it was prominently covered in newspapers. The *China Daily* prominently reported quoting me, 'The virus doesn't kill hundreds of thousands at a thunderous stroke, and it doesn't provide vivid television pictures, he said during the Seventh International Congress on AIDS in Asia and the Pacific in Kobe, Japan. Rather, it is a silent tsunami'. The same quote was picked up by *Los Angeles Times* from distant United States.

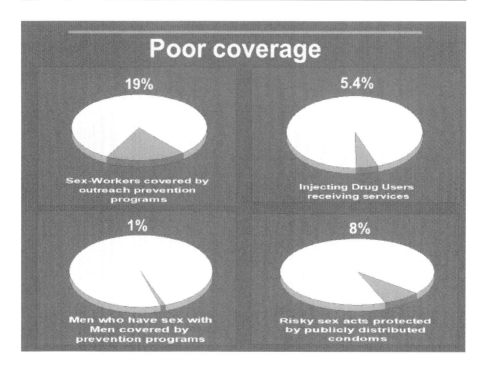

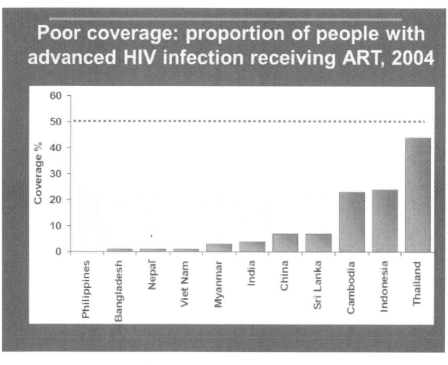

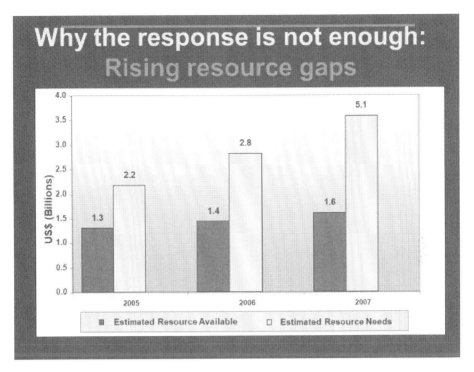

Figure 5: *My Presentation at Kobe ICAAP–Asia Pacific overview of the epidemic and response, July 2005.*

The clear and unambiguous regional picture presented by UNAIDS appealed to the civil society participants and helped establish the credibility of the RST as a regional rallying force for AIDS activism. A tradition was also established that the UNAIDS RST would be the first speaker in future ICAAPs presenting an evidence-based picture of the regional response and setting the agenda for the conference.

STRENGTHENING THE SYSTEMS IN RST

An immediate task after joining the RST was to strengthen the systems in the office and promote a healthy work environment by establishing cordial working relationship between the international and national staff. The UNAIDS regional office was just set up merging the two intercountry units in Thailand and India, and was facing teething problems with personnel getting adjusted to the new job requirements. Staff transferred from India was facing problems in getting adjusted to a new environment they were not feeling comfortable in the initial stages. I met old colleague Swarup Sarkar, who helped me in understanding the office systems and processes. The staff was divided into two broad groups (1) the programme staff or P staff consisting mostly internationals and (2) the general staff or G staff consisting Thai nationals. It did not take me long to realise that the big difference in working conditions and pay structure between the two or the gap, G-a-P as it used to be called between the G and P staff, was affecting the work of the unit. It was a period of transition and there was a lack of clarity and appreciation of each other's role across the organisation. Everyone had an allotted job description and worked in silos towards that.

Transition from a senior secretary level position in government of India to a regional UN job in a foreign country was also a personal challenge for me. My Executive Secretary Watchareeporn Kulpisitthicharoen and I had initially faced difficulty in understanding each other's English! I was used to giving dictations on shorthand in government offices in India, a system which did not exist in UN organisations. I struggled typing out notes on the computer but got used to it in a short time. Paper work was much less in UN system than what I used to have in the Government of India. The Thai staff was very accommodating and tried to put me at ease in the office. Swarup helped me to find a decent accommodation on Sukhumvit Road in the central Bangkok district.

I addressed the issue of morale of the staff first as I believed it was affecting the organisation the most. I met each individual staff member and tried to understand their area of work and related problems. I had done a complete reallocation of work and clearly delineated the roles of the P and G staff. I had done away with the earlier practice of holding separate programme meetings with P staff. All the members of RST staff were invited to the weekly programme meetings which helped in team building. We had organised the first staff retreat in December 2005 at Khao Yae, an hour's distance from Bangkok, and allowed the staff to freely interact with each other. A facilitator was invited to moderate the group sessions. There was a 360-degree evaluation of the director in my absence and the facilitator gave me an extremely positive feedback. I was happy I was moving in the right direction and carried on with my minor management reform in the office.

GLOBAL TASK TEAM AND DIVISION OF LABOUR AMONG UN COSPONSORS

Around this time certain important developments took place in UNAIDS headquarters to improve AIDS coordination among the cosponsors of the joint programme. A global task team (GTT) was established by governments, civil society, United Nations agencies and other multilateral and international institutions to develop a set of recommendations on improving the institutional architecture of the AIDS response, particularly streamlining, simplifying and harmonising procedures and practices to improve the effectiveness of country-led responses and reduce the burden placed on the countries. The GTT was cochaired by Lennarth Hjelmåker, Sweden's special ambassador on HIV/AIDS, and Michel Sidibe, UNAIDS Director of Country and Regional Support. In its 14 June report, the GTT on Improving AIDS Coordination Among Multilateral Institutions and International Donors (GTT) called on the UNAIDS secretariat to lead a process with UNAIDS cosponsors to clarify and cost a UN system division of labour for technical support to assist countries to implement their annual priority AIDS action plans.

The process began by agreeing on 17 broad areas of UNAIDS technical support and identifying a 'Lead' and 'Main Partner' organisations in each of these areas. Each of the UNAIDS organisations would lead in at least one technical area. This information is presented in a Technical Support Division of Labour matrix (see Table 4).

■ Table 4: UN TECHNICAL SUPPORT DIVISION OF LABOUR MATRIX

TECHNICAL SUPPORT AREAS	LEAD ORGANISATION	MAIN PARTNERS
STRATEGIC PLANNING, GOVERNANCE AND FINANCIAL MANAGEMENT		
1. HIV/AIDS development, governance and mainstreaming, including instruments such as PRSPs, and enabling legislation, human rights and gender	UNDP	ILO, UNAIDS Secretariat, UNESCO, UNICEF, WHO, World Bank, UNFPA
2. Support to strategic, prioritised and costed national plans; financial management; human resources; capacity and infrastructure development; impact alleviation and sectoral work	World Bank	ILO, UNAIDS Secretariat, UNDP, UNESCO, UNICEF, WHO
3. Procurement and supply management, including training	UNICEF	UNDP, UNFPA, WHO, World Bank
4. HIV/AIDS workplace policy and programmes, private-sector mobilisation	ILO	UNESCO, UNDP
SCALING UP INTERVENTIONS		
Prevention		
5. Prevention of HIV transmission in healthcare settings, blood safety, counselling and testing, sexually-transmitted infection diagnosis and treatment, and linkage of HIV prevention with AIDS treatment services	WHO	UNICEF, UNFPA, ILO
6. Provision of information and education, condom programming, prevention for young people outside schools and prevention efforts targeting vulnerable groups (except injecting drug users, prisoners and refugee populations)	UNFPA	ILO, UNAIDS Secretariat, UNESCO, UNICEF, UNODC, WHO
7. Prevention of mother to child transmission (PMTCT)	UNICEF	WHO, UNFPA
8. Prevention for young people in education institutions	UNESCO	ILO, UNFPA, UNICEF, WHO
9. Prevention of transmission of HIV among injecting drug users and in prisons	UNODC	UNDP, UNICEF, WHO, ILO
10. Overall policy, monitoring and coordination on prevention	UNAIDS Secretariat	All Cosponsors

SCALING UP INTERVENTIONS

Treatment, care and support

11. Antiretroviral treatment and monitoring, prophylaxis and treatment for opportunistic infections (adults and children)	WHO	UNICEF
12. Care and support for people living with HIV, orphans and vulnerable children, and affected households.	UNICEF	WFP, WHO, ILO
13. Dietary/nutrition support	WFP	UNESCO, UNICEF, WHO

Addressing HIV in emergency, reconstruction and security settings

14. Strengthening HIV/AIDS response in context of security, uniformed services and humanitarian crises	UNAIDS Secretariat	UNHCR, UNICEF, WFP, WHO, UNFPA
15. Addressing HIV among displaced populations (refugees and IDPs)	UNHCR	UNESCO, UNFPA, UNICEF, WFP, WHO, UNDP

MONITORING AND EVALUATION, STRATEGIC INFORMATION, KNOWLEDGE SHARING AND ACCOUNTABILITY

16. Strategic information, knowledge sharing and accountability, coordination of national efforts, partnership building, advocacy, and monitoring and evaluation, including estimation of national prevalence and projection of demographic impact	UNAIDS Secretariat	ILO, UNDP, UNESCO, UNFPA, UNHCR, UNICEF, UNODC, WFP, WHO, World Bank
17. Establishment and implementation of surveillance for HIV, through sentinel/ population-based surveys	WHO	UNAIDS Secretariat

The framework was expected to help in streamlining technical support from the UNAIDS cosponsors under a single technical support plan.

While the general principle of division of labour among cosponsors and secretariat was sound, I could see an operational challenge in the area of support for scaling of prevention interventions. In Asia Pacific, majority of infections were occurring among the key populations of sex workers, drug users, transgenders and MSM. But these groups can't be segregated into watertight compartments in the sense that a sex worker may also inject drugs and an MSM can also be a male sex worker. It was necessary to address prevention as an integrated issue for all the key populations. This was the core agenda for the UNAIDS secretariat, which was eminently suited to take on this responsibility. Under the division of labour, prevention among the key populations was divided among UNFPA (for sex workers) and UNODC (for drug users). Prevention among MSM and transgenders was later given to UNDP. Except for the global coordinators of these three organisations who had experience and expertise in allotted areas, other functionaries down the line were not exposed to the allotted work or communities active in that area. And the UNAIDS secretariat was given the task of coordinating the work divided between three large UN organisations which was not an easy task. I tried to raise this issue in one of the SMTs but understood that it was part of the secretariat–cosponsor issues which needed to be 'amicably' settled.

To take on this additional responsibility the three UN organisations had to carry on an extensive exercise to strengthen their offices at the regional and country level by recruiting experts in the respective areas of work. Many of the new recruits lacked the community-level experience that was so essential for their functioning. I could see that the standard and quality of technical support the country programmes needed in these three important areas of prevention was not forthcoming to the desired level from the UN system. The UNAIDS secretariat had to often step in to fill the gaps. It might be controversial to say this, but the fragmentation of technical support in the important area of prevention among key populations between designated UN agencies and weak coordination among them to deliver as one was an important contributory factor for prevention losing its focus in national AIDS programmes. This was true not just for Asia Pacific region but across the prevention agenda in other regions also.

REGIONAL UN TASK FORCES

At RST Asia Pacific, we tried to overcome this problem in operationalising the framework by constituting a Regional Directors Forum for AIDS with the Regional UNDP Director as chair and the RST Director acting as convener. Constitution of regional level task forces with representatives of communities, the country programme managers and the lead UN agencies under the Division of Labour was also initiated to bring in multisector involvement in prevention of HIV among key populations. This was later extended to migrants through a coordinating mechanism jointly chaired by the UNDP and UNAIDS RST and to sex workers with UNFPA and RST jointly chairing it. These regional mechanisms helped the communities in interacting with the lead UN cosponsors with UNAIDS RST playing the role of a facilitator and coordinator. To that extent I was happy to see that the objective set by the GTT to bring in a framework for coordinated technical support to countries was set to be achieved in the Asia Pacific region.

The first such regional task force (RTF) on drug users was constituted based on a community interaction organised on the sidelines of the Kobe ICAAP. A regional mechanism on drugs and HIV was in existence since 1997, but got re-energised after UNAIDS RST and UNODC Regional Centre for Asia Pacific (RCEAP) assumed joint ownership. Akira Fujino, the UNODC regional representative for South East Asia, and Gary Lewis for South Asia were close allies in the task force. AusAID a prominent donor member initiated a regional programme for harm reduction in South East Asia which had a larger drug user community.

The RTF had three thrust areas in its mandate: (1) advocacy for gradual elimination of compulsory detention of drug users, (2) promotion of harm reduction programmes for mitigation of drug-related harm and (3) making ART services available to HIV-positive drug users through community involvement.

Abolition/phasing out of compulsory drug-detention centres (CDDCs) in East and South East Asian countries was a major priority for the RTF.

Adeeba Kamalruzzaman et al estimated that 'the region had more than a 1000 centres incarcerating over 235,000 drug users for periods ranging from 6 months to more than three years ostensibly for the purpose of drug treatment and rehabilitation. In the name of treatment the drug users were subjected to physical abuses like torture, denial or inadequate provision of medical treatment and unspecified period of detention. Because of denial of treatment many of these centres report high rates of HIV and Hepatitis-C (HCV) prevalence'.[7]

The high relapse rates showed that this method had failed to curb the problem of drug use in these countries with no lessons learnt. Despite introduction of harm-reduction programmes such as needle and syringe exchange (NSP) and oral substitution therapy (OST), the practice of compulsory detention continued. In the next few years the RTF actively pursued abolition of drug-detention centres with the governments of China, Vietnam, Malaysia and Indonesia. By the time I left the RST in 2009, Malaysia decided to phase out compulsory detention centres. Vietnam was actively considering phasing out CDDCs and was not admitting new cases for detention. The move to call for abolition of CDDCs picked up momentum and in March 2012, 12 United Nations entities issued a joint statement calling for the closure of compulsory drug detention and rehabilitation centers. The existence of such centers, which were operating in many countries for the past 20 years, raised human rights issues and threatened the health of detainees, including through increased vulnerability to HIV and tuberculosis (TB) infection.

On the community front, the 'First Consultation on the Prevention of HIV Related to Drug Use' was held in January 2008 in Goa, India. I attended the event which provided a platform for Asian drug-user community to hold a regional consultation and develop the Goa declaration which said 'If Asian and the Pacific governments, civil society, health care providers and other stakeholders are serious about halting the HIV/HCV epidemic, purposeful attention and action must be given to ensure evidence-based and non-oppressive approaches to address the needs and extremely high vulnerability of the IDU population in Asia and the pacific. Policies on drug control need to be harmonised with HIV and HCV prevention, treatment, care and support efforts and standards of services for harm reduction would also be required in order to have an enabling environment for sustainable service delivery'.

The Goa consultation resulted in the birth of the first regional community organisation of people who use drugs–the Asia Pacific Network of People who Use Drugs (ANPUD) in October 2010.

We followed a different approach to evolve a regional mechanism for MSM and transgender community. Naz Foundation and India's NACO together wanted to organise a regional meet of MSM community in Delhi and asked us to support the move. Venue was the same Ashoka Hotel which refused accommodation for an MSM meeting 6 years ago! The consultation, named 'Risks and Responsibilities' held from 23 to 26 September 2006, brought together 380 delegates from governments, policymakers, donors, researchers, grassroots and community-based organisations (CBOs) from 22 countries across the Asia Pacific region and 8 other countries around the world. Several donor agencies namely Department for International Development (DFID), the World Bank, Canadian International Development Agency (CIDA), Swedish International Development Cooperation Agency (SIDA), Australian Agency for International Development (AusAID) and some international nongovernmental organisation (INGOs) for example HIV/AIDS Alliance provided funding and technical support. UNAIDS RST provided technical support for the consultation. I cochaired the opening ceremony with Shivananda Khan from Naz Foundation. Nafis Sadik was a keynote speaker. The 3-day deliberations brought several important players including parliamentarians, researchers, government representatives apart from the large number of MSM and transgender community members.

One of the principle outcomes of the consultation was formation of 'pan Asia/Pacific regional network of organisations and institutions to generate region-wide coordinated advocacy for policy change, social justice, rights, and an equitable allocation of public resources for HIV interventions, care, treatment and other services. This network will ensure that MSM and transgender (TG) issues remain on the HIV agenda in Asia and the Pacific and at all relevant national and regional HIV conferences and meetings'.[8]

The MSM community quickly followed up on the recommendation from the consultation and formed an alliance in July 2007 named as the Asia Pacific Coalition on Male Sexual Health (APCOM). We provided initial funding from RST budget for meeting the operational expenses. Funding support was also provided by Hivos and Naz Foundation International (NFI). Geoff Manthey, the RPA from RST actively worked with the community to complete the registration process. Over the next few years APCOM emerged as a strong regional network, representing a diverse range of interests to advocate and prioritise HIV issues that affect MSM and transgender people.

An important offshoot was the decision that transgender people should have separate projects run by CBOs catering to specific transgender needs. Donors and governments should make funding support available for such activities. This decision had enabled the TG community to form their own organisations instead of getting subsumed in the overall MSM agenda. In India community leaders including Laxminarayan Tripathi, Akkai Padmashali, Abeena Aher and Simran Shaikh played a key role in bringing to centre stage the long neglected social and economic issues plaguing the transgender community and establishing their identity as equal citizens in India.

In working with the regional organisation for sex workers, we had limited success. Our efforts to constitute a regional UN task force for sex workers did not bear fruit despite sincere attempts from the RST and UNFPA, the lead agency. Both UNFPA and the RST found it very challenging to establish a working relationship with the Asia Pacific Network of Sex Workers (APNSW), the regional network which was already functioning in the region. It was not until 2010, the year after I left the RST, that the first regional consultation for sex workers could be organised.

ASHODAYA SAMITI AND ACADEMY

While searching for possible collaboration with sex worker organisations, we came across the Ashodaya Samiti in Mysore, India, which was successfully running a learning site for sex workers from various states in India. Established in December 2005, and formally registered as a Society, the organisation comprised of female, male and transgender sex workers, and strove for the advancement of sex workers in Mysore, Mandya, Kodagu, Hassan, and Chikmagalur districts of Karnataka. It was implementing a project funded by Bill and Melinda Gates Foundation through the University of Manitoba. After an evaluation of its work in imparting skills to sex workers, we decided to recognise it as a learning site for sex workers in the region by forming Ashodaya Academy. The Academy was formally launched by Michel Sidibe, Executive Director, UNAIDS and the Chief Minister of Karnataka in Bangalore in 2010, a few months after I left the RST.

Since then, the Ashodaya Academy has been a laboratory of innovative teaching methods tailored to the local context and the recipients of the training. It uses a mix of field- and classroom-based training to transfer the learnings from its experience in building and nurturing a community-led organisation and spearheading an HIV-prevention model. Learnings from these training programmes were translated into a curriculum that has been shared through peer-to-peer learning processes through Ashodaya workers serving as mentors and trainers. This curriculum has since been used in various countries in the Asia Pacific region. Sushena Reza Paul, Director of the Academy and a public health professional working as Assistant Professor in the University of Manitoba, Canada, provided excellent leadership to the academy during the formative years.

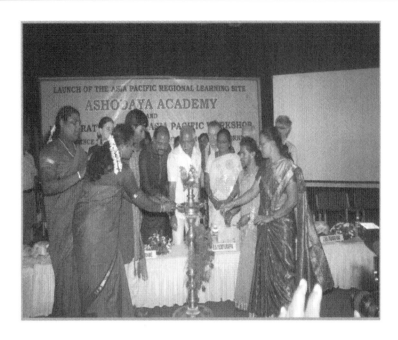

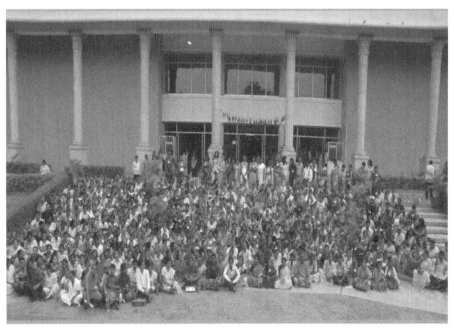

Ashodaya Academy inaugurated by Chief Minister, Karnataka, and Michel Sidibe, EXD UNAIDS

UNIVERSAL ACCESS BY 2010

As we were trying to work on these partnerships at regional level, leaders of the world met at the September 2005 World Summit at United Nations General Assembly (UNGA) as a follow-up to the Millennium Summit and resolved 'to create a more peaceful, prosperous and democratic world and to undertake concrete measures to continue finding ways to implement the outcome of the Millennium Summit and the other major United Nations conferences and summits so as to provide multilateral solutions to problems in the four following areas: Development, Peace and collective security, Human rights and the rule of law and Strengthening of the United Nations'.[9]

One of those commitments was for a massive scaling-up of HIV prevention, treatment, care and support with the aim of coming as close as possible towards Universal Access (UA) by 2010 for all who need it. This move towards UA was endorsed by the UNGA and also by the African Union and the G8 countries.

The Outcome document issued at the end of the summit declared 'Developing and implementing a package for HIV prevention, treatment and care with the aim of coming as close as possible to the goal of universal access to treatment by 2010 for all those who need it, including through increased resources, and working towards the elimination of stigma and discrimination, enhanced access to affordable medicines and the reduction of vulnerability of persons affected by HIV/AIDS and other health issues, in particular orphaned and vulnerable children and older persons'.

To take this resolution forward, UNAIDS organised seven regional consultations on UA. The Asia Pacific consultation was held from 14 to 16 February 2006 in Pattaya, Thailand. Twenty countries from Asia Pacific participated in the consultation hosted by the Thai Ministry of public health. Civil society played an active role and made a strong case for an enhanced role at national and regional levels. Delegates recommended equal representation and decision-making power to civil society in national policy and decision-making bodies and suggested that capacity building and strengthening human resources for civil society should be included in the national budgets. Michel and some of his colleagues from Geneva attended the consultation. That was the first large meeting of country representatives held after I joined the RST and provided an opportunity to interact with the national programme managers and health secretaries from the region. The RST UNAIDS assumed a leadership role in shaping the recommendations from the consultation which were presented in the plenary on the final day. The regional representatives of the UNAIDS cosponsors were present in full strength and witnessed a rare unanimity among the country representatives in accepting UNAIDS leadership at regional level to steer the agenda of UA in AIDS response. From RST, Swarup Sarkar and Sun Gang supported by Nana Kuo provided technical support to the country representatives for finalising the recommendations.

We could, in the consultation, evolve consensus among the countries on some bold and pathbreaking recommendations from the consultation, such as:

➢ Creation of a regional AIDS watchbody that would oversee the commitments of governments, civil society, donors and others concerned in the AIDS response.

➢ Creation of a regional mechanism for price negotiations and procurement of drugs and diagnostics. Delegates strongly recommended increasing the production capacity of generic manufacturers within the region.

➢ Establishment of a regional technical support mechanism to support country-level programmes.

These recommendations found place in a global report on moving towards UA for consideration at the UNGA in May-June 2006.

AIDS DATA HUB FOR ASIA PACIFIC REGION

Since my association with India's national programme, I considered data and strategic information as key to motivate governments to launch cost-effective prevention interventions. I found that capacity to build and analyse strategic information was not available in adequate measure across the countries in Asia Pacific region. After the meeting with ADB in Philippines in 2005 we identified this as a critical need and included it in the MOU to establish the first-ever one-stop online data hub providing comprehensive and easy-to-access HIV and AIDS data in Asia and the Pacific regions. In August 2005, after intensive efforts the UNICEF Asia Pacific regional office and the RST signed an agreement for co-funding the initiative.

The Evidence to Action Initiative as it was known initially was a partnership between the ADB, UNAIDS, UNICEF and WHO. The aim was to provide user-friendly data on most at-risk population groups, women, children and young people, disaggregated by age and sex. It would also probe the provincial and district-level situation where data was available, and provide updates on the prevalence, behaviours and national responses.

The Data Hub as it was named later, was initially located in Mahidol University in Bangkok, but was shifted to UNICEF and later to RST with dedicated staff to perform the functions of data mining, maintaining regional and country profiles, maintaining a web portal and providing request-based customised products to users. It started providing technical assistance for modelling and estimations, policy scenarios and impact analysis.

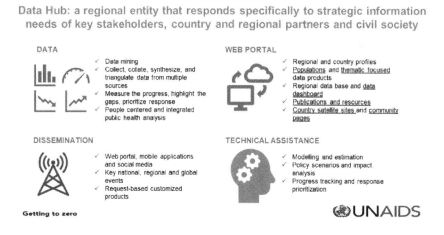

Figure 6: AIDS Data Hub–scope of work.

In course of time, the Data Hub and the strategic data and information provided by it helped to prioritise interventions on those populations who were most at risk, and achieved a high level of service coverage and behavioural change to halt the spread of HIV in the most cost-effective way.

The Hub evolved with the changing and emerging needs of AIDS response and became a well-known regional entity that specifically responded to the strategic information needs of regional, national and community partners. In the past 10 years the Asia Pacific AIDS Data Hub became one of the best practice models within UNAIDS itself. To this day the RST Data Hub functions as a unique technical resource for providing strategic information to users, a facility not seen in any other region.

REVISION OF REGIONAL HIV ESTIMATIONS

On the epidemiological front, there were exciting developments on estimation of national prevalence in Asian countries which had a strategic impact on the regional estimates of HIV prevalence. Four countries revised their national estimation process by using the national level family health surveys that captured a more realistic prevalence of HIV among the general population. The most significant of them came from India which carried the largest prevalence of 5.2 million.

A field study done by a group of researchers from Hyderabad on the HIV estimations in Guntur district of Andhra Pradesh led to the conclusion that the estimated figures based on sentinel survey data could lead to an overestimation of numbers. The researchers led by Lalit Dandona from PHFI cited important reasons for the over estimation, such as addition of substantial HIV estimates from STI clinics in the sentinel surveillance method, referral of HIV-positive and suspect patients by private practitioners to public hospitals including antenatal clinics and a preferential use of public hospitals by lower socioeconomic strata that had higher HIV prevalence. The study concluded that 'application of conservative correction factors derived from the Guntur study reduced the 2005 official sentinel surveillance based HIV estimate of 3.7 million 15–49 years old persons in the four major states to 1.5–2.0 million, which would drop the official total estimate of 5.2 million 15–49 years old persons with HIV in India to 3–3.5 million.[10]

These results came at a time when the third round of National Family Health Survey (NFHS 3) was conducted by the Ministry of Health and Family Welfare. For the first time the results brought out HIV seroprevalence figures among adult population in urban and rural areas of the country. These levels were markedly below the antenatal clinic (ANC) data on which NACO was relying for estimation of national HIV prevalence. In 2006, improved data were available from multiple sources. Sentinel surveillance among ANC women was expanded covering nearly every district in the country, allowing better geographical representation with adequate data for each state to undertake state-specific estimations. The NACO could utilise this opportunity to validate the surveillance data and assumptions used in the estimation process. A group of experts consisting of Arvind Pandey from ICMR, D.C.S. Reddy from WHO, Peter Ghys from UNAIDS and others reexamined the national HIV estimates in the background of these developments and improved data from NHFS 3. To make the estimations compatible with international standards, the WHO/UNAIDS-recommended Workbook 9 and Spectrum10 were adopted for the 2006 HIV burden estimation.

The revised estimate of people living with HIV/AIDS (PLHA) in the population of all ages stood at 2.5 million (uncertainty bounds 2.0-3.1 million). Adult prevalence decreased slightly from 0.45% (range 0.36-0.58%) in 2002 to 0.36% (range 0.29-0.46%) in 2006.The results were published in a study conducted by Arvind et al.[11] The numbers recommended by the group of experts were officially accepted by NACO and UNAIDS and the estimates of earlier years were also modified using the new methodology.

Downward revision of prevalent figures for similar reasons was also done in Cambodia. The Cambodian Demographic Health Survey (CDHS), conducted in 2005, included assessment of HIV infection status. The results of the survey, which was based on a household sampling methodology, were released by the National Institute of Statistics, Ministry of Planning, in April 2007. The estimated national prevalence of HIV infection among adults aged between 15 and 49 was 0.6%. These results differed substantially with the findings of the HIV sentinel survey (HSS) that was conducted by the National Centre for HIV/AIDS, Dermatology and Sexually Transmitted Diseases (NCHADS) in 2003, which estimated the national prevalence of HIV infection among pregnant women as 2.2%. National estimate of people living with HIV infection based on this survey was 1.9%. In Thailand and

Vietnam, similar adjustments were done on population-based surveys instead of sentinel survey data, but the national HIV prevalence figures did not undergo a correction like in India or Cambodia. The regional estimations for HIV prevalence underwent a revision due to these developments, bringing down the number of HIV-positive persons to 5.4 million from 8.3 million.

We were looking for an appropriate regional forum to make an announcement about the revised regional HIV data and the reasons for the downward revision. The 8th ICAAP in Colombo planned for August 2007 provided the best opportunity to speak on this issue.

8TH ICAAP 2007–COLOMBO

Kobe to Colombo was an onward journey with several positive developments. Sri Lanka wanted to host the 8th Conference in 2007 and the organisers announced it at the Kobe Conference in 2005. David Bridger, our focal point for ICAAPs was moved to Sri Lanka as the UCC, which made it easier for us to plan the event. The Sri Lankan Government provided full support and wanted the conference being held in South Asia after a long interval to succeed. The Health Minister, Nimal Siripala De Silva, was personally involved in ensuring a smooth conference. It was a matter of prestige for the country to provide a secure environment at a time when it was deeply embroiled in a separatist agitation by Liberation Tigers of Tamil Eelam (LTTE) militants. I travelled to Colombo and met the UN security officials along with David for a detailed assessment of the security situation. While the general security environment in the country was tense, they did not perceive any threat for a health-related meet such as ICAAP. The Sri Lankan Government officials and the organisers of ICAAP briefed us about the security arrangements being planned for the safety of the delegates. After satisfying ourselves about the arrangements and the commitment of the host government, we decided to go ahead with the event.

The conference, held from 19 to 22 August 2007, attracted over 3000 delegates despite the adverse security environment and the negative publicity that went with it. On the first day, I presented an overview of the epidemic as I did in Kobe, 2 years ago. I wanted to utilise the opportunity to speak on the revision of regional HIV prevalence and the reasons for such a revision. I announced that the regional HIV prevalence stands at 5.2 million because of revisions carried out in the national figures by India and Cambodia. I wanted to steer clear of any avoidable controversy on numbers and went at length explaining the change in estimation methodology and drop in numbers. This helped us in later years to adopt a consistent approach in publication of numbers from Asia Pacific region.

I had to caution that 'It's extremely important to understand this point, because it tells us that the key factors that underpin our battle against the AIDS epidemic have not significantly changed...... even in the revised estimates, nearly 6 million people in the Asia-Pacific region are likely on present trends to be infected with HIV by 2010. Half a million people could still be becoming infected every year and more than 300,000 people could still be dying every year, more than the number of people killed by the Asian Tsunami of 2004'.[12]

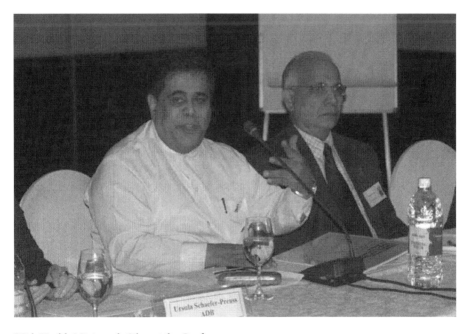

With Health Minister de Silva at the Conference

The conference was able to focus on the key issues of stigma, lack of access to services and declining political commitment to AIDS programmes in the region. The community participation was visible with the launch of the newly constituted APCOM, the regional organisation of MSM community. Some nontraditional donors such as ADB, Japan Bank for International Cooperation (JBIC) and AusAID actively participated in the conference.

The local organising committee, under the leadership the three cochairs Sheriffdeen, Weerakoon, and Sujatha Samarakoon and the conference coordinator Kamanee Hapugalle, were applauded for accomplishing a great task. The UA targets were adopted by most of the countries. Although prevalence rates remained low across the region, rates of new infections were rising in number of countries namely PNG, Vietnam, Indonesia, Nepal and Bangladesh. At the closing ceremony, I stressed that the stigma and discriminatory laws still pose serious obstacles in the region and demanded that national policies focus on the 'forgotten faces of the AIDS epidemic'. There was renewed emphasis on the need for continued activism. We seemed to be losing our way in pursuing it as an effective weapon in our fight against AIDS. We cannot afford to lose our activism–and I used Justice Edwin Cameron's definition: we are all activists in this response. It became clear in a number of sessions that conflict and unstable political conditions could disrupt national AIDS programmes in conflict zones and divert resources from health and social programmes to the military. But even in difficult settings it was possible to deliver services and people have rights to services. Donors should be encouraged not to withdraw from such environments. Asia Pacific donors attending the congress were asked to commit to play a larger role in the region.

The Government of Sri Lanka had tried hard to avoid any hitch while carrying out the events of the conference, but at the end of the conference the health minister reacted to a comment from Jeff O'Malley, the rapporteur general, on non-availability of condoms at the conference. The health minister commented 'I don't want people to think I brought all these people here (for the congress) to promote lesbianism and homosexuality. There are many nice women and handsome men in Sri Lanka'. This utterance by a senior political leader of the host government was resented by some participants. But for us, the organisers and UNAIDS team, it was a big relief that the event passed off smoothly without any problem. The large Indonesian delegation at the venue welcomed the participants to the next ICAAP in 2009 at Bali.

REGIONAL MANAGEMENT MEETINGS

As a part of the decentralised structure of management, regional management groups were established with RST programme staff and UCCs for providing the opportunity to the field staff to discuss programmatic priorities with senior management and assist with the changed management process by facilitating interaction on key operational/management issues relating to the decentralised structure. On June 10 and 11, 2005, we organised the first Regional Management meeting in Bangkok. Peter and Michel with some senior management staff from Geneva attended the meeting. All the UCCs from the region participated in the meeting.

The first such structured interaction between the field staff and senior management proved extremely productive and provided an opportunity for the executive director to get a firsthand feedback of the country-level responses in 15 countries where UNAIDS established a strong presence. Peter was happy with the outcome and complemented the RST for taking the lead in organising the regional group meetings.

I later thought it would be necessary to use the forum to establish strong linkages with national programmes at the regional level by inviting senior-level programme managers from countries for a structured interaction with the UNAIDS family from countries, regions and headquarters. In April 2008, we organised the first such interaction of the forum with national programme managers and senior health officials from countries. Dr. Nafsiah Mboi, Secretary General of NAC from Indonesia, Dr. Francisco Duque III, Principal Secretary Health from Philippines, Dr. Teng Kunthy from NAC Cambodia along with senior programme managers from other countries attended the meeting and enriched the discussions. It was extremely productive and there was an immediate demand to conduct that interaction periodically–at least once in 6 months. Nafsiah Mboi immediately responded by inviting us to hold the next such interaction at the ICAAP Bali in Indonesia.

During my tenure of 5 years I attached great importance to the half-yearly regional management meetings (RMMs) and got positive support from both Peter and Michel. These meetings helped the senior management team in Geneva enormously to understand the field-level issues the country programme managers and the civil societies have to contend with in responding to the AIDS challenge in the region.

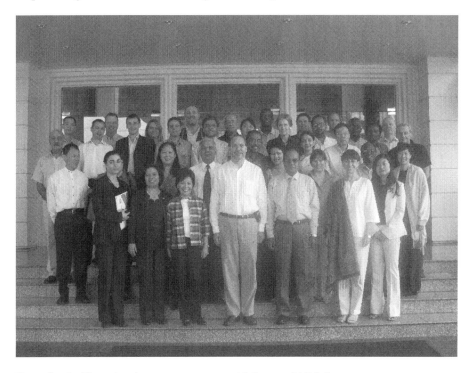

Happy family: The regional management team with Peter and Michel.

COMMISSION ON AIDS IN ASIA

After attending the first RMM of the RST in Bangkok in June 2005, Peter, in a one-to-one discussion, expressed his concern on lack of political support at the highest level for AIDS programmes in Asia Pacific region which was hindering the progress. He came up with the idea of setting up an independent group of experts drawn from development sector to take a deep dive into the dynamics of AIDS response, and identify the developmental challenges the countries of the region would face if AIDS was not effectively controlled. The political leadership in the region should be made aware of the damage the AIDS epidemic would cause to the economies of the countries not just in terms of health costs but the deep economic impact of losing productive sections of population to AIDS. He asked me to suggest the name of a well-known development economist from India who could head such a group. I thought about several persons and ultimately suggested the name of Dr. Chakravarthi Rangarajan, the Chairman of the Economic Advisory Council to the PM of India. Dr. Rangarajan was a distinguished development economist of India and served as the Governor, Reserve Bank of India (Indian equivalent of the US Federal Reserve System) and Governor of the state of Andhra Pradesh. He was appointed as the Chairman of the Economic Advisory Council to the PM Dr. Manmohan Singh with a Cabinet rank after the UPA government took office in 2004. The challenge was to make him agree to take up the assignment because of his busy engagement with the PM. I travelled to Delhi to meet him and explained the purpose of setting up the group. He asked why he was being asked to join the group without any experience of working in AIDS programmes. I explained to him that the group will have a mix of AIDS and non-AIDS experts and UNAIDS wants it to be chaired by an economist with development background. He was enthusiastic but wanted a thorough briefing on the regional profile of the epidemic and the response. Events moved quickly and we got his approval to chair the committee. We then went on to select the other members to make the body fairly representative across the region. The members came from diverse background but the common trait among all of them was their deep commitment to address the AIDS challenge in the region.

The following personalities joined the group which was named as 'Independent Commission on AIDS in Asia Pacific':

➢ Nerissa Corazon Soon Ruiz, Congresswoman from Cebu, the Philippines

➢ Tadashi Yamamoto, President for Japan Center for International Exchange (JCIE), Japan

➢ Wu Zunyou, Director of National Centre for AIDS and STD Control and Prevention in Chinese Centre for Disease Control and Prevention, China

➢ Mahmuda Islam, Professor of Sociology in Dhaka University, Bangladesh

➢ Tim Brown, Epidemiologist and Senior Research fellow in East West Centre, Hawaii, United States

➢ Rajat Kumar Gupta, Senior Partner Worldwide, McKinsey and Company, United States

➢ Frika Chia Iskander, Coordinator of Women's working group in APN+, Indonesia

➢ Marie Bopp Dupont, Pacific Island AIDS Forum, French Polynesia

I acted as the Member Secretary of the Commission which was established in June 2006.

But in the first meeting itself we faced a hurdle as one of the members from Pacific, Marie Bopp Dupont, expressed doubts about the effectiveness of a composite body for Asia and Pacific. She rightly pointed out that Pacific region had special problems and needed a separate group to address them. Peter and Rangarajan agreed with this approach and we immediately reconstituted the Commission only for Asia and started our work. Marie Bopp opted out but promised to get into the Pacific body as and when it was constituted. In RST, Swarup, Sun Gang, Cho Kah Sin, Nana Kuo from the RST and a new intern Nalin Siripong formed the secretariat for the Commission work. The Commission was given 18 months to submit its report.

For the next 18 months my time was heavily drawn into the AIDS Commission work. But the complexities of the epidemic and significant gaps in strategic information to understand its dynamics were evident to the Commission right from the beginning. The Commission wanted two research initiatives (1) on the long-term projection of the progress of the epidemic and (2) on the medium and long-term impact of AIDS on societies and economies. Tim Brown from East West Centre, agreed to undertake the task of making projections on the numbers based on the Asian Epidemic Model (AEM) his institute had developed. Anita Alban, an AIDS researcher from University of Copenhagen, was entrusted with the work of cost-effectiveness study and Ross Mcleod, who earlier worked in ADB, did the resource needs assessment study. We initiated the work in November 2006 by dividing it into four tracks, Policy, Epidemiology, Resource needs and Community involvement. In January 2007, we conducted a policy options workshop where experts from all the four tracks and individual specialists were called to provide various policy options for combating the epidemic. This consultation proved to be extremely useful for the Commission to examine number of policy options and decide upon the most cost-effective and impactful from a civil society perspective. Rangarajan was keen that the role of the communities who are at the centre of the epidemic should be clearly defined. About 600 individuals and community organisations were contacted and in-depth interviews were conducted with key activists. The Commission held sub-regional consultations in Dhaka and Manila with community representatives and government officials. Informal meetings were held with political leaders, administrators, AIDS researchers, civil society partners and senior UN officials.

By October 2007, we assembled the first draft of the report which was discussed over 2 days in a full Commission meeting in Beijing. Peter attended the meeting as an observer and, true to his role, did not make any intervention. At the end he told Rangarajan that he was excited about the report and looking forward to its completion. The report was finally ready by January 2008 and sent for printing.

I was personally very happy with the outcome, a report that clearly defined the epidemic characteristics in Asia and forecasted its progression with and without interventions. The Commission proved with evidence that the Asian epidemic is distinctly different from the African one and a one size fits all strategy will not work. The global classification of the HIV epidemic as low, concentrated and generalised did not express the actual nature and dynamics of the epidemic. The Commission wanted a new classification to be worked out and adopted according to the predominant risk behaviours and their relative contribution to the epidemic. In the interim, four epidemic scenarios were presented: latent, expanding, maturing and declining epidemics for Asia. An attempt was made to quantify the number of people who are vulnerable to the epidemic out of the large population of 3.1 billion in the region. The Commission identified this number as 75 million men who indulge in multipartner sex and 50 million women who were their sexual partners. A smaller number of 10 million sex workers and equal number of IDUs and MSM were at the core of the epidemic and most at risk of getting infected. The cumulative number may appear small compared to the population of the region but large enough to create tremendous pressure on resources for treatment if a sizable section among them get infected. The Commission's emphasis on prevention addressed this very risk of uncontrolled epidemic if a business as usual approach continues in the region. In a resurgent epidemic this number can shoot up to a million new infections every year. In a contained epidemic with strong interventions the number could drop down to as low as 100 thousand. The choices before governments were clearly identified in the report.

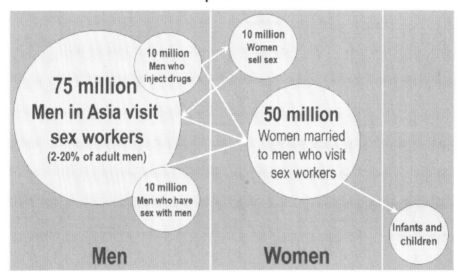

Figure 7: Size of populations vulnerable and at risk of HIV infection.

For the first time the economic impact of Asian epidemic was examined in great detail. The Commission concluded that there would be marginal impact on the gross domestic product (GDP) and longevity in Asia unlike in Africa where it was estimated as substantial. The real impact would be on government and household budgets with precious resources drawn away from priority development programmes to AIDS control to meet the ever-increasing treatment costs and on prevention of growing number of new infections. The studies had shown that it would be wiser to invest in prevention interventions among key populations as they were the most cost-effective. This prioritisation came under challenge with agencies working on youth, migrants and other sections of general population arguing for larger commitment of resources to programmes addressing them. But the per capita costs of these interventions proved to be much higher than the key population-focused programmes and the Commission decided to prioritise programmes for key populations in a limited resource setting. Only in a fully funded programme could all interventions be taken up without bothering about priorities and cost-effectiveness.

The Commission therefore presented two scenarios, one with full funding and another with limited resources. Resources for full response were estimated as $6.1 billion per year which was a tall order. In a limited resource setting, the region would need at least $3.1 billion per year to halt and reverse the epidemic to achieve the target set by MDG by 2015. But the countries were investing only $1.2 billion per year at that time which was not enough to bring substantial reduction in new infections, to provide treatment to the infected population and to mitigate the impact of the epidemic. With a focused prevention package, the Commission was confident that in a period of 12 years (2008-2020) cumulative number of new infections would come down by 5 million, the number of people living with HIV by 3.1 million and AIDS-related mortality by 40% by provision of ART.

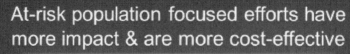

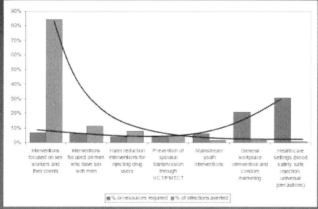

Figure 3.9: Comparison of prevention interventions, according to distribution of resources and percentage of new infections averted, 2007-2020
Source: Redefining AIDS in Asia: Crafting and Effective Response

Commission on AIDS in Asia – Projections and Implications   16

Cost of a Priority Response – high impact

Interventions	Total Cost (millions USD)	% of total
High-impact prevention	$1,338	43%
Treatment by ART	$761	24%
Impact mitigation	$321	10%
Programme Management	$363	12%
Creation of an Enabling Environment	$359	11%
Total	$3,143	100%

Average total cost per capita ranges from $0.50 to $1.70, depending on the stage of the epidemic.

Commission on AIDS in Asia – Projections and Implications   18

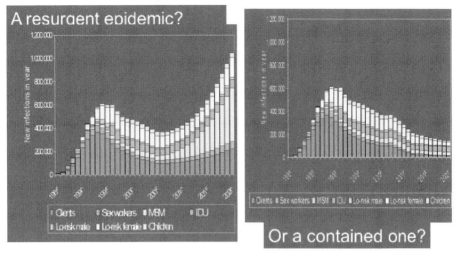

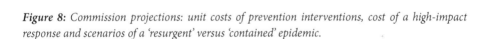

Figure 8: Commission projections: unit costs of prevention interventions, cost of a high-impact response and scenarios of a 'resurgent' versus 'contained' epidemic.

The Commission laid strong emphasis on creation of an enabling environment to ensure success of the HIV-related interventions. Repeal of laws that enshrine HIV-related discrimination, especially those that regulate labour market, the workplace, access to health care and insurance, educational and social services and inheritance rights for women was recommended. Countries were advised to constitute 'AIDS watchdog bodies' to monitor HIV-related discrimination in various settings.

The Commission strongly felt that AIDS activism and civil society advocacy alone could sustain AIDS response in Asia for a long time. To secure this, proactive policies need to be adopted to support communities to organise themselves and to forge partnerships with media, health care providers, government officials and other CSOs.

The 230-page report carried a technical annex which contained all the technical papers, studies and projections made for arriving at the report. The Commission's recommendations, 14 on policy, four each on programme, strategy and implementation under three broad categories–prevention, treatment and impact mitigation and three on governance issues were meant for all the major stakeholders in the AIDS response.

We wanted a formal launch of the report in a highly visible event. But before that we wanted to apprise the Programme Coordinating Board (PCB) of UNAIDS about the report even though it was the work of an independent Commission. Peter agreed to include it in the agenda for the PCB in Chiang Mai, Thailand, in April 2008. Rangarajan and I along with a few commission members travelled to Chiang Mai to attend the technical session where the report was presented to the appreciation of all participants. Unexpectedly, the Thai delegation objected to certain parts of the report containing the Commission's assessment of the current response of Asian countries and how they were falling short in making a major impact. The Commission, based on evidence, felt that Thailand's response was quite advanced and reflected strong leadership and resolute execution during the earlier stage of the epidemic. However, prevention strategies did not reflect the need for harm-reduction programmes even when HIV prevalence among IDUs stayed at a level of 30% for one decade as per the report of HIV surveillance in December 2007. Shifts in political commitment were therefore assessed as medium in 2006 while they were rated as high in 2001. In the main PCB session, the Thai delegates continued to vehemently oppose these observations in the report and did not allow a formal approval of the report by the Board despite overall support from all other country delegates. For the sake of consensus, the Board finally decided to 'take note' of the report and asked the countries to take follow-up action. The objections of the Thai delegation were taken as recorded.

I was very keen that even though it was a regional report it should have a global launch at UN Headquarters in New York. We decided to approach UN Secretary General Ban Ki-moon and were quite elated when he agreed. In June 2008, the report was launched by him in UN headquarters, New York, in the presence of the permanent representatives of number of Asian countries. Rangarajan the chair, members of the Commission and Peter Piot participated in the launch. While releasing the report the SG has said 'As Secretary-General and as an Asian, I am particularly moved to have this chance to contribute to a full and honest discussion about the epidemic in Asia — a discussion which has not always been forthright or open enough in the past'. Describing the report as 'exceptionally topical and timely', he cautioned that 'Several countries are off track on Millennium Development Goal number 6 — halting and beginning to reverse the spread of HIV/AIDS by 2015. Meanwhile, among Asians aged between 15 and 44, AIDS has become the single largest cause of workdays lost and of deaths related to disease. We are seeing the beginnings of a vicious circle, posing a threat to economic growth and social resilience and leading to more and more infections. This compels us to act immediately and unflinchingly to stop the circle turning its deadly wheel until it spins out of control'.[13]

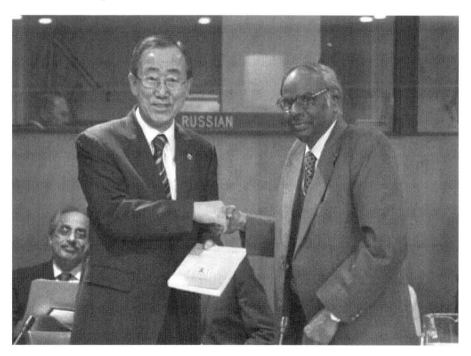

Prof. Rangarajan, Chair of the commission, with the Secretary-General Ban Ki-moon at the launch

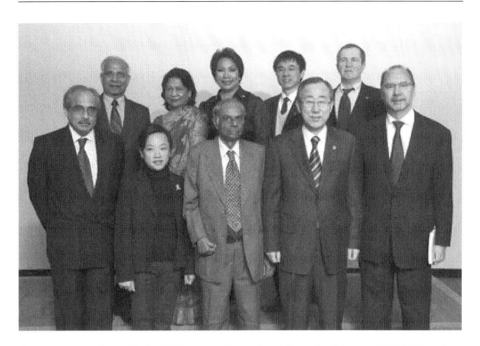

Commission members with the UN Secretary-General and Executive Director of UNAIDS at the launch

It was a fitting climax to our 18 months of hard work, and true to our expectation the report received excellent media coverage and reviews. The Commission members were invited in the evening by Asiatic Society for a community launch at their office in New York.

Back in the region, we followed up with country-level launches in Cambodia, India and Vietnam and received enthusiastic response from political leaders. Prime Ministers, Manmohan Singh in India and Hun Sen in Cambodia attended the meetings and appreciated the recommendations of the Commission. Country-level dissemination was also done in Bangladesh, Nepal, Vietnam, China and Philippines.

In many ways the report of the independent Commission on AIDS in Asia was a pathbreaking one. It strongly laid emphasis on prevention of new infections among so many competing priorities, often driven by technical agencies working in those areas. It proved that preventive interventions among the most at risk populations are the most cost-effective and would give value for money invested. Resource needs were not only quantified but arranged on a graded scale of response. The AEM made a bold prediction that by 2020 large number of infections will occur among the MSM communities which had later proved to be true. The country-level buy-in for the report was exceptional. Many countries had taken the recommendations on board while formulating their national strategic plans.

An important development during the Commission work from 2006 to 2008 was the rapidly changing political scenario in Thailand. The chair, Dr. Rangarajan, visited Bangkok to attend a consultation in September 2006. On September 19, I invited him and his wife, Mrs. Haripriya Rangarajan, to my residence for dinner. The Indian Ambassador in Thailand was also among the invitees. After the dinner when the Rangarajans were ready to leave, the ambassador received a call on his mobile. He came back and announced that there was an army coup in Thailand and PM Thaksin Sinawatra was deposed. Rangarajan had to postpone his return to India by a day and I could not attend office the next day as the entire Rajdamnern Avenue was blocked for civilian movement. The UN heads of agencies met at a location outside the UN building and were planning for a prolonged stay outside. Fortunately, access to the building was restored within a couple of days and Bangkok returned to normalcy without any incident. We all heaved a sigh of relief. But for the next few years Thailand plunged into political uncertainty with military and civilian rule alternating frequently. The area in front of the UN building became the scene of civilian demonstrations for opposing political groups and work was disturbed frequently. But the demonstrations remained mostly peaceful and we even used to enjoy the evening music played by the demonstrators to entertain themselves! But the political uncertainty continued to haunt Thailand for quite some time since that coup which took place after 15 years of constitutional governance.

PACIFIC COMMISSION

By October 2007, we finalised the report of the Asia Commission and it was time to keep our commitment to constitute a separate Commission for the Pacific region. We secured financial support from UNAIDS and started the work with all sincerity. Tracy Newbury, the RPA from Australia who joined us in 2006 was taken into the team because of her familiarity with the region. AusAID and New Zealand Aid Programme (NZAID) showed keen interest in the work and provided financial support. Dr. Langi Kavaliku, former Deputy PM of Tonga, was approached to chair the Commission and seven more members from various Pacific countries were inducted into the Commission. I acted as the member secretary to this Commission also.

We had an immediate setback to our work after the first meeting of the Commission in Nadi, Fiji Islands. In December 2007, Langi Kavaliku died in a traffic accident in Tonga. We faced a crisis of leadership but got the Deputy Prime Minister of Samoa Misa Telefoni Retzlaff as the new chair, and continued with our work. It helped enormously to have him as the chair as he was the AIDS Champion and Health Minister in his country from 1996 to 2001 and spoke at number of international fora. Other members of the Commission were:

➢ Maire Bopp Dupont, an AIDS activist from French Polynesia and Chair of the Pacific Islands AIDS Foundation,

➢ Dame Carol Kidu, Minister of Community Development, Government of PNG

➢ Satish Chand, School of Business, University of New South Wales, Australia,

➢ Rob Moodie, Professor of Global Health at Nossal Institute for Global health at the University of Melbourne, Australia,

➢ Hitelai Polume Kiele, Attorney General and acting Secretary of Justice, PNG,

➢ Warren Lindberg, Group manager Public Health Operations, Ministry of Health, New Zealand

The biggest challenge the Commission faced apart from the sheer logistics of Pacific islands was the inadequacy of data relating to AIDS epidemic in the region. Time series for surveillance data and basic demography of vulnerable populations were not robust. Data on sexual risk behaviour for relevant populations was also inadequate. We attempted to strengthen the evidence base by sponsoring eight research studies which included the future trends of the epidemic and the economic impact of AIDS. A unique one was on the role of churches in the response in PNG. We commissioned two surveys on the perception of people from the Pacific on HIV. We worked closely with the nascent HIV-positive peoples organisations through the Pacific Islands AIDS Forum headed by Maire Bopp.

Like in Asia Commission, field-level consultations were organised in PNG, Samoa, Solomon Islands, New Caledonia and Fiji. I attended the consultations in PNG, Samoa and Fiji. The logistics in Pacific were too daunting for me to cover all the consultations.

The region covers an immense geographical area comprising countries with varied geographical diversity and highly mobile populations. HIV was first reported in 1984 and since then in all the countries and territories except three, Niue, Pitcairn Island and Tokelau. As per UNAIDS estimates about 81,000 people were infected with the virus by 2006 with PNG accounting for 90% of the infections. This proportion shot up to as high as 99% by 2008. All the risk factors such as low condom use, high and accelerating STI rates, lack of sex education and a high degree of population mobility were present in the region. The predominant mode of transmission of HIV was through unprotected sex. Commercial and transactional sex was a major source of HIV vulnerability. The stigma associated with high-risk behaviour was present in equal measure in Pacific society as in mainland Asia. Women comprised majority of reported cases of HIV with PNG diagnosing 14,500 women as against 12,500 men in 2007. If PNG was excluded, the MSM constituted with 33%, the second largest segment of HIV notifications.

It goes to the credit of the leadership of the region that the Pacific leaders acted early to support efforts to mitigate the risks and vulnerabilities and maintain low levels of infections in the region. Even PNG which had all the risk factors favouring a hyper spread of the epidemic such as in sub-Saharan Africa had not witnessed that abnormal growth due to quick handling of the situation by the political leadership. But poor quality of health services across the region restricted the capacity of governments to provided HIV and STI services. More than $77 million could be mobilised for HIV programmes in the Pacific but the cost of implementation of services was also high in the region because of logistical challenges. The dependence on external resources for AIDS programmes impacted the sustainability of the response. The limited absorptive capacity of the countries also made it hard to utilise even the limited resources available to them. Between 2003 and

2005, only 63% of GFATM grants were disbursed and less actually utilised. In PNG only 24% of allotted HIV budget could be spent by the National AIDS Council Secretariat.

As we progressed with the work, we realised that Pacific islands, with the possible exception of PNG, and Fiji would not be able to sustain a standalone programme for AIDS control. The islands were too small to access external resources nationally for HIV-related programmes. The two alternatives possible for them would be building a strong HIV component into the health sector plans or becoming part of a regional HIV plan where funds could be accessed by regional bodies such as the Secretariat of Pacific Community (SPC) or the Pacific Islands Forum (PIF). Coordination of multisectoral responses did follow the principles of 'three ones' in many of the island nations. But the Commission felt that there was no need to establish standalone mechanisms for small nations and the processes can be integrated into national health systems.

Civil society organisations flourished in the Pacific region and strengthened engagement with the communities vulnerable to HIV. But the Commission felt that openness in matters of sexual behaviour and identities in Pacific societies would reduce HIV-related stigma and discrimination.

In finalising the report, the Commission advocated for an OPEN strategy as the way forward for the regional response to HIV/AIDS which stands for

➤ OWNERSHIP of the epidemic at all levels of society.
➤ PARTNERSHIPS to develop integrated response.
➤ EMPOWERING and ENABLING environment.
➤ NETWORKING to share experiences and outcomes.

The Commission made 26 recommendations under the five broad categories of leadership, legislation and enabling environment, civil society, strategic planning and implementation, resources and aid effectiveness. The 135-page report was pathbreaking in nature and the first of its kind to comprehensively address the HIV/AIDS problem in the Pacific region. The Commission completed its work within the assigned time frame of 12 months. There was a general feeling that the UN SG should be approached to launch this report also and it was a pleasant surprise for us when he agreed to do it.

I travelled to New York with fellow members of the Commission to participate in the launch of the Commission report. We had a major scare when the consignment carrying printed copies of the report to New York went missing! With the help of UNAIDS New York office we got sufficient number of copies printed within 24 hours in New York, in time for the launch function. On 2 December 2009, the report was launched by SG Ban Ki-moon in New York; the last month of my stay as RST Director in UNAIDS. Permanent representatives of Pacific countries, Michel Sidibe, the new Executive Director of UNAIDS and members of the Commission attended the launch. The SG in his address had remarked,

'Responses to AIDS in the Pacific must be based on an understanding of the region's peoples, cultures, beliefs and practices. This report takes just such an approach. It weaves together the story of HIV in 22 geographically and culturally diverse countries. We now have a much more complete picture and clear recommendations for action'.

He cautioned that 'In countries with large populations, even several million HIV infections can seem like drops in a bucket. But where populations are small, as in the island nations of the Pacific, infections in the hundreds or thousands can translate into high prevalence rates – with devastating impacts on individuals, families, communities, economies and even security' and urged the countries, donors, UN and civil society to work together to contain the epidemic and its potential impact on the people of the region.

The UNAIDS also commented that 'The Commission's Report is the first document to synthesize regional and country information on epidemiology, risks and vulnerabilities, and financing and coordination of the AIDS response. Issues of rights and civil society as well as the impact of AIDS on health are also highlighted'.[14]

For me it was a great moment of fulfilment coming at the end of my 5-year tenure as Regional Director UNAIDS. As member secretary of both Asia and Pacific Commissions, I contributed to the launching of two pathbreaking reports on the AIDS epidemic in the region. It was a unique distinction for us to get both the reports launched by SG Ban Ki-moon, who demonstrated his love for the region by his active involvement.

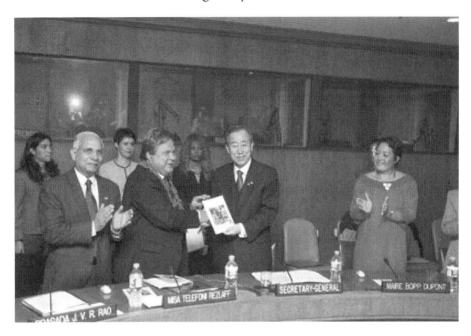

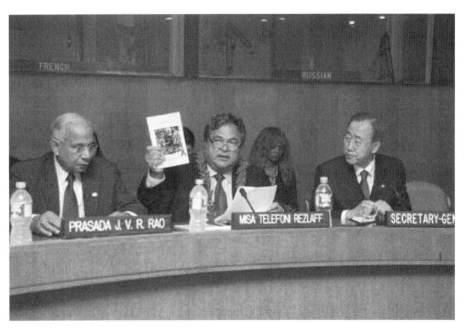

Launch of the Pacific Commission Report in UN headquarters, New York

Like the Asia Commission we also wanted the event to be followed up with country-level launches to generate ownership of the report. Steve Kraus, my successor as RST Director, followed up with launch of the report in PNG on 11 March 2010, where it was presented to Sir Paulias Matanaem, Governor General of PNG. This was followed by launch in Samoa on 22 April 2010, by Tuilaepa Lupesoliai Sailele Malielegaoi, the PM of Samoa. In Fiji, the report was handed over to President Ratu Epeli Nailatikau and representatives of the Pacific Regional organisations on 26 April 2010 by Commission Chair, Misa Telefoni Retzlaff. Steve was gracious to invite me to the Fiji launch where I met President Ratu Epeli who praised the efforts of the Commission and provided full support to its recommendations.

As we were going through the work of Pacific Commission, there was a change of leadership in UNAIDS. Peter Piot who steered the organisation for 14 years after it was established had retired in December 2008. In the 14 years of his leadership, Peter converted a fledgling organisation into the most successful and visible joint UN programme. He was a rare combination of a scientist, a strategist, a programme leader and above all a great visionary. I really missed him in that role but drew satisfaction that someone like Michel Sidibe, who by that time was elevated as Deputy Executive Director, succeeded him. Michel was already known as the leader in waiting and it did not take us long to get adjusted to the transition.

THE aids2031 CONSORTIUM

One of the initiatives Peter started before he left UNAIDS was the establishment of an aids2031 consortium to take a fresh look at the future of AIDS. By 2031, the world would mark the passage of 50 years of the AIDS epidemic from the time the first case was reported in 1981. The international consortium of partners included nine thematic working groups on various thematic topics which included a group on countries with rapid economic transition (CRT) focusing on China, India, Malaysia, Vietnam, Indonesia and Thailand. Peter wanted me to act as the co-convener of this group along with Prof. Myung Hwan Cho from South Korea. I was also made a member of the global steering committee which met periodically to monitor progress of working groups' work. Smriti Aryal, Regional Programme Advisor (RPA) in the RST, provided secretarial support to the working group.

This work enabled us to take a deep dive into the special characteristics of AIDS problem in the newly emerging economies of Asia. These six countries will go through major demographic, economic and social transformation by 2031. Economic transformation will be key; Gross National Product (GNP) will be double in all the six countries, economies will shift from agricultural base to manufacturing and services. Population density will increase and rapid urbanisation will be seen in all the six countries, with a large majority of populations living in urban areas. Social and cultural values and norms will rapidly change and there will be increased interaction and mixing of different ethnicities, classes and culture.

The group held periodic meetings and finalised its recommendations by April 2009. The group felt that with rapid economic development, the per capita health care spending will increase in all the six countries, creating more fiscal space for HIV prevention and treatment. But fiscal space will not automatically provide policy space as political leadership will not be prioritising AIDS programmes in a sustained manner until 2031. Rural-urban migrants will continue to emerge as a key vulnerable group. MSM and transgender communities will evolve as key vulnerable communities. IDU will continue to be one of the main modes of transmission and risk factors in some of the rapid transition countries. Economically driven 'traditional' notion of sex work will continue to flourish as large portion of poor women will continue to sell sex and male clients will continue to be large. Sex will be generally more accessible, with information technology (IT)-enabled services making access to sex easier and anonymous.

In the recommendations the group stressed on the increasing role of governments in the CRT countries as they would become more powerful with economic advancement. All partners will need to use AIDS as an opportunity to bring about wider social sector reforms–decriminalise sex work, same-sex relationships and other forms of legal reform. The group felt that there will now be a greater support from the progressive mainstream societies to the cause of human rights. It will be absolutely important to continuously draw on these progressive elements of the society to join hands with the community leaders and civil society partners in the fight against AIDS in all the CRT countries, more so to empower communities through broader social reform.

The group considered that we should win the battle at the intermediate level if we want to contain the impact of the epidemic by 2031 and felt that the next 10 years would be crucial in the fight against the virus.

The recommendations of the working group on CRT countries were taken on board in the final report of the aids2031 consortium which was launched in February 2011 at the Nelson Mandela Foundation in South Africa, a year after I left the RST. Peter Piot, then the Director of the Institute of Global Health at the Imperial College London, cochaired a panel at the launch and explained the key findings and recommendations of the consortium. The over-arching message was that the world needs to come to terms with the fact that AIDS is not over, not by any measure. 'Sharply reducing the number of new infections and AIDS deaths by 2031 requires new ways of thinking about AIDS and responding to the challenges that the pandemic poses. It requires new prevention and treatment tools; sound policies to optimize the effectiveness of programs; innovative approaches to AIDS financing; the creation of strong and durable capacity in countries; transition from a focus on individuals to one that views communities as critical fulcrums for success; and management practices to maximise efficiency and effectiveness.'[15]

The report concluded that the pandemic was not going away, but its magnitude and severity can be dramatically curtailed if the global community brings the seriousness of purpose to this problem it deserves.

FOLLOW-UP ON AIDS COMMISSION REPORT: INTIMATE PARTNER TRANSMISSION OF HIV

The new evidence the AIDS Commission for Asia brought out on the estimated number of men and women who are vulnerable to the infection brought a new dimension to the approach on preventing the epidemic. When 75 million men and 50 million women are vulnerable to the virus because of sexual transmission, the agenda of prevention needs to be expanded to cover these sections in the general population. The projections made by UNAIDS for 2020 showed that low-risk women and MSM constitute the largest segments at risk of getting infected. Mobile men with money are two to four times more vulnerable than nonmobile men. They and their intimate partners, men and women had to be brought into the focus for preventive interventions.

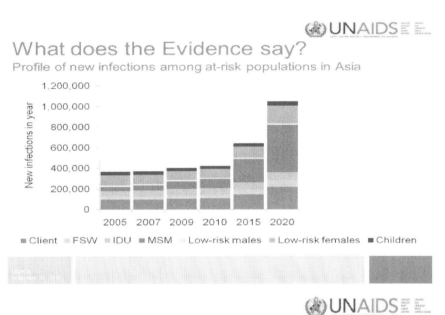

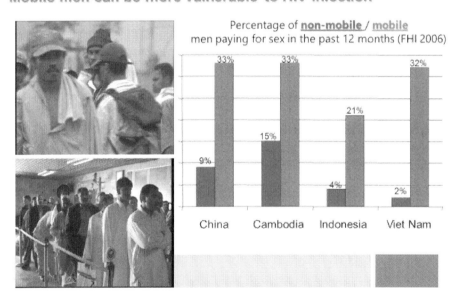

Figure 9: Infection trends in Asia and vulnerability of mobile men.

To follow-up on AIDS Commission report, we undertook a new initiative in the RST to focus on preventive interventions for intimate partner transmission (IPT) and advocate with countries to integrate IPT prevention into their sexual and reproductive health (SRH) programmes. To protect female partners of men at risk, preventive interventions among migrants and mobile populations should include their female sexual partners. Vulnerable women and their male sexual partners should be identified with structural interventions. The sexual and reproductive needs of MSM, sex workers, IDUs and PLHAs need special attention in national SRH programmes.

9ᵀᴴ ICAAP BALI, INDONESIA

We once again decided to choose a regional forum to highlight the IPT issue and the 9ᵗʰ ICAAP in August 2009 at Bali, Indonesia, provided an excellent platform. The Bali ICAAP held from 9 to 13 August was one of the largest in attendance and an enormous success.

Bali ICAAP also took place in the shadow of terrorist attacks in Jakarta, and President Susilo Banbang Yudhoyono, in his inaugural speech went out of his way to declare his government's firm commitment to ensure a peaceful conference despite the terrorist attacks. 'I assure you that the recent attacks in Jakarta will not change the fact that Indonesia is a stable, peaceful democracy grounded on freedom, pluralism and tolerance, just as you see and feel here in Bali. I also wish to commend all of you for keeping this Conference on schedule in Bali, Indonesia despite the terrorist attacks in Jakarta last month. This is the way it should be. There is no better way to send a message to terrorists than to demonstrate that they cannot and will not deter us from freely and fearlessly living our lives and keeping our way of life' he said.

On the AIDS problem, he spoke openly saying that it was one of the greatest public health challenges. He called the response as a glass half full, conveying that a lot of work needs to be done to build on the successes. He spoke about the challenges Indonesia was facing in Papua province which may get into a low-level generalised epidemic if timely action was not taken. 'I think it is the consensus of this conference that we see the glass half full, not half empty. ….. In Indonesia, we also see the glass as half full…… The

Asian Epidemic Modeling (AEM) projections show that if we do not act now, in ten years there could be two million Indonesians living with HIV. That is a scary prospect', he warned.[16]

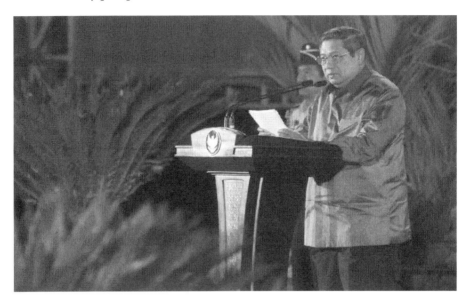

President Yudhoyono inaugurating Bali ICAAP

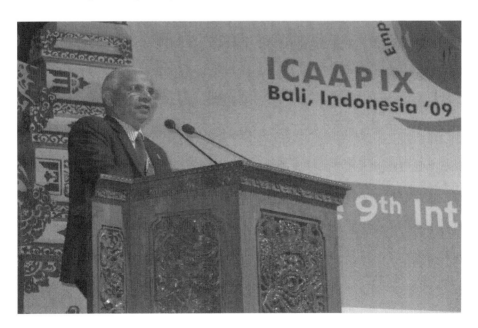

Presenting the regional profile of AIDS response at the plenary

Nafsiah M'boi, Secretary of the National AIDS Commission, was the co-organiser of the Conference and provided exceptional leadership. She was a source of great strength to the national AIDS programme, having worked for long years as a civil servant in the government and later in WHO. The Conference was a rallying point for communities who participated in large numbers. The Joint UN programme on AIDS was represented by almost all the 11 cosponsors who had thrown their weight behind the Conference.

Together we had organised a symposium on HIV and IPT during the Conference with participation of Nafis Sadik, the UN SG Special Envoy on AIDS, Women of Asia Pacific Network of people living with HIV (WAPN+), the United Nations Development Fund for Women (UNIFEM), the United Nations Population Fund (UNFPA) and the International Centre for Research on Women (ICRW). The key message from the symposium was that understanding and addressing HIV transmission among intimate partners was one of the most complex, difficult and sensitive areas but it was also the key to dealing with the rapidly rising HIV epidemic in the region and may even be the key to turning it around. At the end a framework was developed to address IPT which included (1) integrating the protection of women into HIV prevention programmes, (2) scaling up of prevention for MSM, IDU, clients of sex workers and stressing on the protection of their female partners, (3) scaling up of prevention among mobile populations and migrants and focusing on protecting their intimate partners and (4) structural interventions for vulnerable women and their male sexual partners.

'Paramount to effective interventions, it is critical for us to have costing that counts and to ensure that women-focused interventions are included and budgeted in national development strategies, plans and programmes and translated into action on the ground'.[17]

In October 2009, I followed up on this message later at the Asia Pacific Conference on Sexual and Reproductive Health and Rights (SRHR) in Beijing. I presented a strong case to expand SRHR programmes to include the needs of populations who were at risk of IPT. I advocated for expansion of the reproductive and child health (RCH) programmes to include male sexual health and pay special attention to the needs of vulnerable women especially those experiencing gender-based violence. Integration of PMTCT programmes into health systems and promoting dual use of condoms were other initiatives needed to address IPT in health care systems.

These two high-profile events enabled us to advocate strongly with governments to keep the interests of women at risk of HIV as a key focus in their national AIDS responses.

Ibu Nafsiah also kept her promise to host a meeting of all the national programme managers from Asia Pacific countries at the ICAAP. We had a long and detailed session where country programme managers freely interacted and shared their experiences and lessons learnt in the national AIDS programmes.

Among my last engagements as Director RST Asia Pacific was attending the high-profile World AIDS Day 2009 event in New York and the launch of the Pacific Commission report by the UNSG on 2 December. I was completing 5 years of very intense and exciting stay in the job which I never thought I would be in. I had an excellent team of technical and supporting staff at Bangkok and a band of highly energetic UCCs in the field. Together, this team worked hard to keep AIDS high on the political agenda of countries. There were enormous challenges but also small victories to celebrate. The doomsday scenario of a runaway AIDS epidemic with high prevalence levels in general population was disproved. No country except PNG recorded a rate of more than 1% prevalence in general population. Even in PNG, thanks to resolute action by the government and participation of communities, there were signs of a slowing down if not stabilisation of the epidemic. Countries such as Thailand, India and Cambodia brought substantial reduction in new infections and were well on the way to reach the MDG of halting and reversing the epidemic by 2015. In the region as a whole, as against 5.2 million infections in 2005, the prevalence in 2010 stood at 5.4 million, the slight increase explained by increasing survival rates of people on ART. New infections registered a substantial drop from 450,000 to 350,000 from 2005 to 2010. AIDS-related mortality decreased from 330,000 to 270,000, nearly 20% drop in 5 years.[18]

Most satisfying for me was the establishment of regional CBOs, APCOM and ANPUD and the regional learning site at Ashodaya Academy for sex workers which helped in filling a vital gap in community empowerment in the region.

As a UN entity, the joint programme had its limitations. It can't take the role of an implementor except in conflict situations or while working in a failed state. It can certainly present the countries the best evidence on the cost of a failed or delayed response as was done very effectively through the work of two independent Commissions for Asia and the Pacific. The problem of scarce resources always acted as a limiting factor to what the RST could do. But we had the satisfaction of putting the resources to the best possible use by focusing on niche areas and following a country-specific approach. Swarup moved to Global Fund as Director Asia and a new area of collaboration between UNAIDS and GF was emerging. The Social Development Division of UN ESCAP got a new Director, Nanda Krairiksh. In my first interaction with her I requested that the regional body should use its convening power to rally the countries in the region for a stronger commitment on AIDS response. But it was time for me to leave all these matters to my successor, Steve Kraus, who as Global AIDS Coordinator in UNFPA was intimately involved in the programme at the global level.

I travelled to Geneva for a debriefling with the Geneva team and to meet Michel Sidibe to bid goodbye. There was a subtle feeler if I would be interested to join in a senior position in Geneva. But I made up my mind to get back to India and told Michel that I did not want to continue with a 9 to 5 routine anymore. He wanted me to work in an Advisory role giving limited time to support him. That was a suitable mechanism and we both agreed to pursue it after my return to India.

In the last RMM held on 15 December 2009, I got a standing ovation from all my colleagues and an affectionate message from Michel who could not attend the meeting. It was followed with a farewell function and a retreat where my colleagues sang and danced to a Bollywood number to show their intense love and affection towards me. I was deeply moved. I had spent 5 years with this dream team and it was time to take leave.

I laid down office at the end of December 2009 and moved back to Delhi as the New Year 2010 dawned upon the world.

REFERENCES

1. United Nations Economic and Social Council. Resolution 1994/24. 1994/24 Joint and co-sponsored United Nations programme on human immunodeficiency virus/acquired immunodeficiency syndrome (HIV/AIDS). Available at: https://data.unaids.org/pub/externaldocument/1994/19940726_ecosoc_resolutions_establishing_unaids_en.pdf.

2. A scaled up response to AIDS in Asia Pacific–UNAIDS 2006. UNAIDS 2005.

3. A scaled up response to AIDS in Asia Pacific–UNAIDS 2006. UNAIDS 2005; Figure 10.

4. A scaled up response to AIDS in Asia Pacific–UNAIDS 2006. UNAIDS 2005; Figure 11.

5. UNAIDS. Intensifying HIV prevention. UNAIDS policy position paper. 2005. Available at: https://www.unaids.org/en/resources/documents/2005/20051205_jc1165-intensif_hiv-newstyle_en.pdf

6. UNAIDS. Joint United Nations Programme on HIV/AIDS & APLF. Asia Pacific Leadership Forum on HIV/AIDS and Development, Act Now: Asia-Pacific Leaders Respond to HIV/AIDS, UNAIDS/APLF, Bangkok, June 2004, 52 pp. Available at: *https://data.unaids.org/publications/external-documents/apfl_actnow_en.pdf*

7. Kamarulzaman A, McBrayer JL. Compulsory drug detention centers in East and Southeast Asia. *International Journal of Drug Policy*. 2015;26(1):S33-S37.

8. Khan S, Bondyopadhyay A, Causey P. Risks and Responsibilities. Final Report. 2006. Available at: https://www.apcom.org/storage/2017/08/Risk-and-Responsibilities-2006-Technical-Report.pdf

9. United Nations General Assembly. 2005 World Summit Outcome. 2005. Available at: https://documents-dds-ny.un.org/doc/UNDOC/GEN/N05/487/60/PDF/N0548760.pdf?OpenElement

10. Dandona L, Lakshmi V, Kumar GA, Dandona R. Is the HIV burden in India being overestimated? *BMC Public Health*. 2006;6:308. doi: 10.1186/1471-2458-6-308.

11. Pandey A, Reddy DCS, Ghys PD, et al. Improved estimates of India's HIV burden in 2006. *Indian Journal of Medical Research*. 2009;129(1):50-58.

12. ICAAP 2007. Plenary Speech by Prasada Rao. 8th International congress on AIDS in Asia and the Pacific. 2007.

13. Ban ki-moon. Asian states must act 'immediately and unflinchingly' to stop AIDS epidemic, says Secretary-General at launch of Commission report: [remarks, on the handover of the report of the Commission on AIDS in Asia, New York, 26 March 2008] / [by the UN Secretary-General]. New York:

UN Dept. of Public Information. Available at: *https://digitallibrary.un.org/record/626409?ln=en*

14. Annual Report 2009. UNAIDS Web site. Available at: https://www.unaids.org/sites/default/files/media_asset/2009_annual_report_en_0.pdf

15. aids2031 2009 Young Leaders Summit. Report of the Consortium on aids2031. 2009

16. Speech of H.E Susilo Banbang Yudhoyono, President of Indonesia at the Opening Ceremony of 9th International Congress on Aids in Asia and the Pacific (ICAAP). 2009;Densapar, Bali. Available at: *https://www.unodc.org/documents/southeastasiaandpacific/2009/08/ICAAP/ICAAP9_SBY_SPEECH_OPENING_09082009.pdf*

17. 9th International Congress on Aids in Asia and the Pacific (ICAAP). HIV and Intimate Partnership Transmission. Symposium Summary. 2009. Bali.

18. Technical Assistance Completion Report. TA 7519-REG: Evidence-Based Advocacy for Fighting HIV/AIDS in Asia and the Pacific: Regional HIV/AIDS Data Hub. 2010. Available at: https://www.adb.org/sites/default/files/project-document/42988/43438-012-tcr.pdf

CHAPTER 4

PLAYING A ROLE ON GLOBAL FRONT (2010-2017)

After returning to Delhi I had to devote my time to settle down in a city I left 5 years ago with many of my old friends and acquaintances moving away from the capital after retirement from the government. Michel quickly followed upon our conversation in Geneva and appointed me as his Special Advisor for the Asia Pacific region. In a region I was familiar with, I was asked to work as a regional advocate for prioritising AIDS programmes and interact with senior political leaders in high disease burden countries and advise the executive director (EXD) on where the response was failing and needed his intervention at political level. As Special Advisor to EXD I was provided with needed support–a place to work in UNAIDS country office in Delhi and secretarial assistance. Denis Braun, the UNAIDS Country Director in India, put me at ease in organising my work. I started living in Gurgaon (now Gurugram), an IT hub on the outskirts of Delhi and was commuting to office as and when needed. For the first time after more than four decades of work life I was experiencing the freedom of not rushing to office in the morning with a 9 to 5 routine. In that role I could organise my routine including working from home and going to UNAIDS India Office only when needed.

GLOBAL COMMISSION ON HIV AND LAW

As I was settling down to the new life and work in Delhi, Jeff O'Malley, Director HIV/AIDS in United Nations Development Programme (UNDP) Headquarters, New York, informed me about establishment of a new global commission on HIV and Law. The legal environment–laws, enforcement and justice systems—has immense potential to better the lives of HIV-positive people and to help turn the AIDS crisis around. Restrictive laws criminalise behaviours of key populations namely sex workers, drug users, men who have sex with men (MSM) and transgender communities and inhibit them from accessing prevention and treatment services. He informed me that UNDP as an important cosponsor of the joint programme and UNAIDS together decided to set up an independent group of experts as a global commission to examine the interface of legal environment and people who are infected and affected by HIV/AIDS. The Commission was expected to analyse existing evidence and generate new evidence on rights and law in the context of HIV and develop rights-based and evidence-informed recommendations. Former President of Brazil, Fernando Henrique Cardoso, was approached to chair the Commission and 14 other members from various regions were proposed as commissioners. Jeff and his deputy Mandeep Dhaliwal were my long-time associates and wanted me to join the Commission to act as its Commissioner Secretary. My work with the two regional commissions on AIDS in Asia and Pacific must have prompted them to make this choice.

The members of the Commission were:
- Former President of Brazil, Fernando Henrique Cardoso (Brazil, Commission Chair),
- Justice Edwin Cameron (South Africa),
- Ms. Ana Helena Chacón-Echeverría (Costa Rica),
- Mr. Charles Chauvel (New Zealand),
- Dr. Shereen El Feki (Egypt, Commission Vice-Chair),
- Ms. Bience Gawanas (Namibia),
- Dame Carol Kidu (Papua New Guinea),
- The Honourable Michael Kirby (Australia),
- The Honourable Barbara Lee (United States),
- Mr. Stephen Lewis (Canada),
- His Excellency Mr. Festus Mogae (Botswana),
- Mr. JVR Prasada Rao (India),
- Professor Sylvia Tamale (Uganda),
- Mr. Jon Ungphakorn (Thailand) and
- Professor Miriam Were (Kenya).

I was quite excited by this unforeseen development but thought it might affect my work in my new role in UNAIDS. When I raised this issue with Michel Sidibe, he considered it as a positive development and encouraged me to join the Commission. He felt that my work with the Global Commission will only reinforce my role as Special Advisor and will not cause any adverse impact. I joined the Commission and was drawn for the next 18 months into another intensive work schedule and travel to different regions and UNDP Headquarters in New York. At the first meeting with Jeff, Mandeep and others in June 2010 in UNDP New York, I shared my experience in working with similar commissions in Asia and Pacific. We discussed several issues including preservation of the independent nature of the Commission, meeting the tight 18-month deadline, holding of regional consultations to ascertain the views of regional- and country-level actors and constitution of a technical advisory group (TAG) to analyse technical data and provide independent advice to the Commission. An e-group was set up to enable close interaction between the commissioners and the secretariat.

The first meeting of the Commission was hosted by the Chair of the Commission, President Cardoso in Sao Paulo, Brazil. The agenda for the Commission work, the timetable for regional consultations and the TAG mandate were finalised. The commissioners got to know each other in that meeting. I was happy to meet Justices Michael Kirby and Edwin Cameron, prominent members of the Commission a decade after my last meeting with them in Delhi as Director of the National AIDS Control Organisation (NACO). Justice Cameron left the Commission on technical grounds after the first meeting.

In February 2011, the regional consultations and TAG meetings started with the first consultation for Asia Pacific organised in Bangkok. Others quickly followed: Trinidad and Tobago for Caribbean in April, Moldova for Eastern Europe and central Asia in May, Brazil in June, South Africa in August, Middle East and North Africa in July 2011 in Cairo and high-income countries of North America and Western Europe in United States in September 2011. The second meeting of the Commission was held in August in Johannesburg along with the regional dialogue for Africa. It was a very intensive and exciting period of 6 months of regional work, I as

Commissioner Secretary was required to attend to. I could not attend the Cairo event but managed to participate in all the others. Commissioners were asked to join the consultations in their respective regions and the Commission chair joined the dialogue in Sao Paulo, Brazil. The Oakland consultation for developed countries was actively supported by Congresswoman and Commissioner Barbara Lee along with her team.

The Regional Dialogues aimed to provide an opportunity for community members to share experiences of legal environments, both enabling and repressive, on their lives in the context of HIV, and to engage in dialogue with experts and representatives from governments and the legal community in the respective regions. Apart from communities, representatives from national programmes, governments, parliament and UN agencies were invited to participate.

For me it was a great opportunity to understand not just the legal environment but the overall AIDS response in various regions and compare them with my Asia Pacific experience. What struck me most was the criminalisation of HIV transmission, which posed a serious threat to treatment access. Willful transmission of HIV by an infected person can normally be addressed under ordinary criminal law of the country and there was no need to enact special laws for this purpose. But I found it most pronounced in Africa. Criminalisation of same-sex relations and sex work were quite prominent in countries that reported a higher prevalence of HIV; clearly establishing the link between HIV and adverse legal environment. Availability of antiretrovirals (ARVs) was another challenge prominently discussed in these dialogues. A new dimension was the push to get new laws on counterfeit drugs enacted in African countries by powerful multinational drug companies to stop manufacturing and import of generic drugs from India, Brazil and other generic drug-manufacturing countries.

The dialogue in Oakland with developed countries was quite an eye opener for many of us. It was not a wellknown fact that high-income countries accounted for vast majority of criminal prosecutions relating to HIV nondisclosure, exposure or transmission. The criminalisation of HIV transmission among the vulnerable communities had a strong racial and minority bias. Many of the community leaders highlighted this aspect in their presentations with clear evidence. Majority of persons arrested/ prosecuted under various criminal laws governing HIV were Afro Americans and Hispanic people in United States and black minorities in Europe and Canada. Many developed countries had rising infection rates among these very populations who were stigmatised and singled out for harsh treatment by the police and law-enforcing authorities. Countries in the region had enacted criminal laws and wherever such laws did not exist, prosecutions were filed under ordinary criminal law. The practice of enacting separate legislation for criminalisation of HIV transmission had apparently been picked up by African countries essentially from this region. In 2010, the United States launched a National AIDS Strategy which called for an end to the criminalisation of HIV transmission and exposure. Number of countries including Norway and Finland had begun a review of legal provisions that criminalise HIV transmission and exposure. In 2001, Portugal became the only European Union (EU) member state to explicitly decriminalise illicit drug possession and use– since then the number of newly reported cases of HIV among people who use drugs has declined substantially every year from 2001 and drug use had not increased.

In December 2011, the third and final meeting of the Commission was held at Geneva to facilitate the attendance of some of the commissioners at the UNAIDS programme coordinating board (PCB) held around the same time. The draft report was ready after taking the comments of TAG members on board. We had an interesting scenario with some commissioners calling for a report that speaks to activists above everyone else and that pushes the envelope on rights and justice. From the opposite perspective, we had some who were very concerned about a potential backlash and wanted the recommendations to be very firmly and rigorously defended with evidence. A third group including me preferred to adopt a more practical approach, calling for a report that speaks to all important stakeholders–political leaders, religious leaders, traditional leaders and a broad base of civil society leaders including activists based on strong field-level evidence.

The December meeting of the Commission was followed by the PCB of UNAIDS. I took the opportunity to update the PCB on the status of the Commission's work.

I asked for PCB's indulgence in answering questions such as the following:

➢ How can we promote 'test and treat' when many countries around the world criminalise people living with HIV?

➢ How can we reach, involve and empower the populations most at risk of HIV when in too many settings, they risk prosecution simply for being identified as sex workers, MSM, transgender people or drug users?

➢ How can women safely seek and benefit from prevention of mother-to-child transmission (PMTCT) services when often they have no legal protection against the risk of gender-based violence that may arise from disclosing their status?

I reminded the PCB that the current opportunities for getting to zero and the current funding crisis made the securing an enabling legal environment all the more urgent. (*My speech at the UNAIDS PCB, Geneva 15 December 2011.*)

As the report of the Commission was getting ready, I was invited to a high-level meeting (HLM) convened by UN Economic and Social Commission for Asia and Pacific (UNESCAP) Bangkok in February 2012 to speak on the work of the Global Commission on HIV and Law as a Commissioner. Representatives from 34 Asia-Pacific countries met from 6 to 8 February at the Asia-Pacific High-level Intergovernmental Meeting on the assessment of progress against commitments in the Political Declaration on HIV/AIDS and the Millennium Development Goals (MDGs). The meeting was convened by the United Nations regional commission to find ways to speed up progress towards an AIDS-free region, including by removing legal and policy barriers that hamper access to HIV services. The meeting endorsed a road map based on greater regional cooperation to fast-track progress towards meeting global commitments on the 2011 Political Declaration on HIV and AIDS and the MDGs. The regional meeting was the first major intergovernmental meeting of its kind after the historic adoption of the Political Declaration on HIV and AIDS by world leaders in June 2011.

After several iterations with suggestions coming from commissioners and TAG members, the Commission report was presented for a final round of discussion through teleconference in March 2012. We ironed out many of the earlier differences. The consensus was that the recommendations had to be universal and should challenge the countries to set a national road map, depending upon the state of the epidemic and the legal environment prevailing in that country.

By March 2012, we had finished with the Global Commission work and as Commissioner Secretary I was happy with the outcome. The Commission was assisted by a strong group of experts in the TAG and an extremely knowledgeable set of professionals such as Tenu Avafia, Brianna Harrison and Emilie Pradichit in UNDP secretariat. It was an exciting partnership with fellow commissioners namely Michael Kirby, Edwin Cameron, Stephen Lewis, apart from the two former heads of state, President Fernando Cardoso from Brazil and President Festus Mogae from Botswana and Congresswoman Barbara Lee from Oakland, United States.

For the launch of the report, the secretariat of UNDP approached the Executive Office of United Nations Secretary-General (UNSG) who indicated that 9 July 2012 would be convenient for the launch. A Global Dialogue with participation of commissioners and some civil society representatives was also planned. We later heard that the Deputy SG Jan Eliasson would do the launch as SG Ban Ki-moon was preoccupied. Michel Sidibe and Helen Clark, Administrator UNDP confirmed their participation. From the Commission, President Festus Mogae, Congresswoman Barbara Lee, Charles Chauvel and I attended the Global Dialogue and the launch of the report. I was a bit disappointed that SG Ban Ki-moon could not attend the ceremony. It would have been a hat trick for me to have the SG launching the three reports of Independent Commissions! President Cardoso joined the dialogue on video and Stephen Lewis joined the morning media conference by telephone. It was an impressive performance by all.

Speaking at the launch of the Commission Report

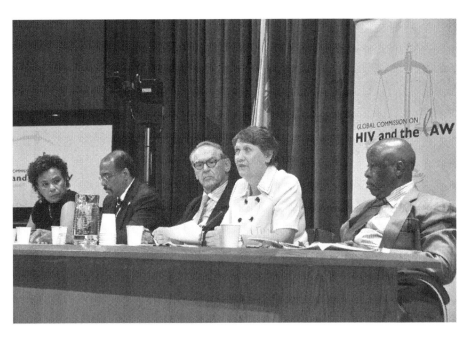

Congresswoman Barbara Lee, Michel Sidibe, DSG, Helen Clark and President Mogae at the launch

We received a great deal of positive response to the report. The commissioners wanted a report that could be used as a tool by civil society in their ongoing campaigning. The feedback from activists around the world had been unequivocal: you have succeeded. Even some of the Commission's most significant sceptics had responded with delight to the report, its analysis and its recommendations. We have also had significant media pick up, particularly in social media, in Africa and in public health-related publications. Interestingly the *Bangkok Post* carried an extremely adverse article criticising the Commission's stand on the issue of sex work and drug use, reflecting a highly conservative viewpoint. President Cardoso and Jon Ungphakorn, the chair and the commissioner from Thailand, promptly issued a rejoinder explaining that it was an independent body which had made the recommendations on the basis of clear evidence and the editorial piece in the newspaper was highly opinionated and not based on evidence.[1]

The report of the Global Commission was quickly followed up with national-level events in many countries in Africa, Asia and Western Europe. UNDP secretariat worked with civil society partners in over 59 countries on Commission follow-up. This included supporting work on HIV-related law review and reform, judicial and parliamentarian sensitisation, national dialogues for HIV-related law reform and HIV-related access to justice programming.

On 4 December 2012, the US National Dialogue was led by Commissioner and Congresswoman Barbara Lee. This dialogue focused on issues of HIV criminalisation and engaged legislators and civil society from the 34 states with problematic HIV criminalisation laws. The Commission report was also launched at the House of Commons in London, United Kingdom. Many Asian countries initiated legal consultations to discuss the Commission recommendations and develop a road map for their implementation. On 1 December 2012, in the World AIDS Day message, SG Ban Ki-moon also highlighted the report of the commission. 'I also urge stronger efforts to eliminate the stigma and discrimination that increase risk for vulnerable populations. The *Report of the Global Commission on HIV and the Law: "Risks, Rights and*

Health" emphasises how outmoded laws, misguided judiciary systems and punitive policing practices – based not on science but on fear and prejudice – fuel the epidemic. We must make information, testing and treatment available to all, so every man, woman and child can enjoy their fundamental right to the medical care and essential services that will end this devastating epidemic' he said.[2]

INTERNATIONAL AIDS CONFERENCE, WASHINGTON 2012

The report and its findings quickly reverberated in another important forum, the International AIDS Conference in Washington held within a few days of launch of the report in July 2012. I spoke at a symposium organised by the Global Commission and UNDP titled 'Global Commission on HIV and Law – A movement for HIV Law reforms' on Commission's recommendations on sex work and drug-use issues. Congresswoman Barbara Lee, commissioners Shireen El Faki and Stephen Lewis spoke on various recommendations of the Commission. The report received wide publicity coming within a few days before the conference.

But the IAC Washington got into a controversial start. Sex workers and drug users were prohibited from travelling to the United States under 'moral turpitude' restrictions. Washington's conference organisers warned that the government officials may use 'various methods' to research travellers' backgrounds. Short-term one-off waivers may be granted, but this was at the discretion of consular officers. When a waiver was granted, it was recorded in the visa system permanently, which activists said could function like a scarlet letter and prevent entry to the United States in future.

Protesting against this arbitrary decision, the sex worker community decided to abstain and hold a parallel conference at Kolkata, India, a few days prior to the Washington meet. I was specially invited to attend the Kolkata meet not just as a commissioner but as someone who was associated with India's national response as Director NACO. In my address I pointed out, 'These two groups [sex workers and drug users] have to be kept central to the global response to HIV, and their absence makes any discourse on HIV and AIDS insufficient and not meaningful. While the IAC in Washington will have a large gathering of AIDS activists, the exclusion of two important communities robs it of the universality of its message............They have been literally forced into organising a separate conference instead of participating in the main event in Washington. It shows that the battle for recognition of their rights is still a long and arduous one, and stigma and discrimination are still the overriding issues for vulnerable communities'.

The Kolkata conference organised under the banner 'save us from saviours', was the largest ever global gathering of sex workers. It was made an official IAC hub and was connected to Washington by video link. It also had its own agenda, with a focus on key freedoms such as the freedom to move and migrate, access to quality healthcare and freedom from stigma and discrimination.

SPECIAL ENVOY TO UNSG ON AIDS IN ASIA PACIFIC

As I was winding up my work as Member Secretary of Global Commission on HIV and Law, I got a message from Michel Sidibe that I should attend a meeting at Mumbai in April 2012 where the SG Ban Ki-moon would be participating in an event connected with 'Every Woman Every Child initiative'–a programme the SG was closely associated with. He also alerted me that there would be an announcement concerning me in the meeting. I could guess what it could be. Nafis Sadik who served as the Special Envoy of the Secretary-General (SESG) for Asia Pacific for little more than a decade wanted to retire and it would be another Asian who had to succeed her. I met the SG at the function organised by Reliance Foundation, a philanthropic organisation chaired by Nita Ambani where he announced my appointment as the next Special Envoy on AIDS for Asia. There was a good assemblage of celebrities including Mukesh Ambani, the head of Reliance group, Noeleen Heyzer, the Executive Secretary of UNESCAP, Health Secretary, Keshav Desiraju, and some Bollywood personalities among others. I felt humbled at this recognition of my work on HIV/AIDS spanning about 15 years starting from 1997 when I had joined NACO to lead India's national response. I thanked the SG at the dinner that followed and pledged my support to his endeavors to make a difference in the global response to AIDS. Michel felt very happy at my appointment and assured me of all support from UNAIDS for my work. I started receiving affectionate greetings from Asia and other parts of the world also. I informed the Global Commission on HIV and Law and received greetings from fellow commissioners, Jeff, Mandeep and other members from the secretariat.

Three other SEs on AIDS were appointed for Eastern Europe and Central Asia (EECA), Caribbean and Africa regions. For some reasons there was a quick turnover of Africa Envoys and finally it was decided that Africa will go without an envoy. Michel Kazatchkine, former EXD of Global Fund to Fight AIDS, Tuberculosis and Malaria (GFATM), and Edward Greene former Assistant Secretary-General (ASG), Human and Social Development at the Guyana-based CARICOM Secretariat were appointed as envoys for EECA and Caribbean regions; the three of us built a close partnership together and worked as a team. The SESG is a UN diplomatic position in the rank of ASG to deal with a set of specific issues and carried an honorary status. The envoy was free to reside at a place within the region and was provided secretarial support from UNAIDS. The UN resident coordinator system provided need-based support especially while undertaking official missions in countries for facilitating meetings with senior political functionaries.

I was happy with this dispensation as I could relocate myself anywhere in the region and chose Bangalore in south India as my place of stay. I shifted from Gurugram to Bangalore in November 2012, a friendly city with a great all-season climate.

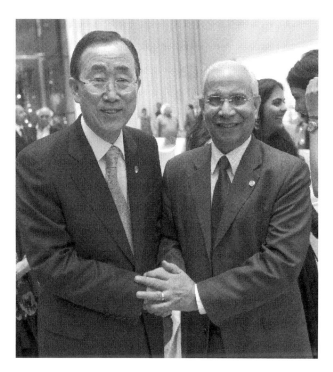

With Secretary-General Ban Ki-moon at the time of my appointment

INTELLECTUAL PROPERTY ISSUES–FOLLOW-UP ON GLOBAL COMMISSION ON HIV AND LAW REPORT

One of the most controversial recommendations of the Global Commission on HIV and Law related to the intellectual property rights (IPR) for pharmaceuticals. Recommendation 6.1 of the Commission reads:

> *The UN Secretary General must convene a neutral, high-level body to review and assess proposals and recommend a new intellectual property regime for pharmaceutical products. Such a regime should be consistent with international human rights law and public health requirements, while safeguarding the justifiable rights of inventors. Such a body should include representation from the High Commissioner on Human Rights, WHO, WTO, UNDP, UNAIDS and WIPO, as well as the Special Rapporteur on the Right to Health, key technical agencies and experts, and private sector and civil society representatives, including people living with HIV.*

The Commission secretariat in UNDP led by Mandeep Dhaliwal and Tenu Avafia initiated an immediate follow-up on the recommendation of the Commission on IPR. The secretariat organised a consultation in New York with experts on IPR issues, representatives of WHO and UNAIDS, government and civil society representatives. I was invited to the consultation in September 2013 as a former commissioner and as the Special Envoy of UNSG. Helen Clark, the administrator of UNDP, Michel Sidibe EXD UNAIDS and my fellow envoys Michel Kazatchkine, and Edward Greene also participated in the event. We had an intensive 2 days of consultation and decided to request the UNSG to constitute a high-level panel (HLP) of experts on the lines of the high-level panel of eminent persons (HLPEP) constituted to help him in defining the post-2015 development agenda. The HLP should be mandated to study and recommend a new intellectual property regime as a part of the post-2015 development agenda with the objective of making available affordable and good quality medicines to global poor. The panel may have representation from important stakeholders such as governments, civil society and experts on intellectual property issues. The UNDP, UNAIDS and United Nations Office of High Commissioner for Human Rights (UNOHCHR) can serve as the secretariat for such a panel which can be mandated to submit its report to inform the discussion in the United Nations General Assembly (UNGA) on post-2015 development agenda. This became necessary as the present TRIPS regime which regulates the availability and affordability of medicines had failed to make life-saving medicines accessible to poor and needy around the world. Lack of access to affordable medicines was one of the principal reasons for the failure of many countries in achieving the health-related MDGs by 2015.

After internal consultations between UNDP and UNAIDS, a communication was finally sent to UNSG on 14 October 2013 by the Administrator UNDP, EXD UNAIDS and UNORHCR requesting him to convene a neutral, high-level body to review and assess proposals and recommend a new intellectual property regime for pharmaceutical products that is consistent with international human rights and public health needs.

The SDG agenda took precedence at that time and the constitution of the Panel was delayed. Finally we three SEs of UNSG on AIDS followed up with a joint letter to the SG in July 2015 renewing the request for constitution of the HLP. The panel was constituted by the SG in November 2015 with a resolution that 'Consistent with the findings and recommendations of the Global Commission on HIV and the Law, and in line with the aspirations articulated in his synthesis report on the post-2015 development agenda and the recently adopted Sustainable Development Goals (SDGs), the UNSG Ban Ki-moon convened a HLP on innovation and access to health technologies'. The panel was cochaired by H.E. Ms. Ruth Dreifuss, former President of the Swiss Confederation, and H.E. Mr. Festus Mogae, former President of the Republic of Botswana. The overall mandate of the HLP was to review and assess proposals and recommend solutions to remedying the policy incoherence between the justifiable rights of inventors, international human rights law, trade rules and public health in the context of health technologies that is impeding access and the right to health for millions.

The work of the panel was supported by an Expert Advisory group 'assembled to provide technical support to the High-Level Panel. The High-Level Panel and its Expert Advisory Group were supported by a Secretariat based at UNDP, New York which will also work with the UNAIDS Secretariat.'

The panel was asked to submit its report to the SG by June 2016 but released its report in September 2016 with a simple yet powerful message: no one should suffer because they cannot afford medicines, diagnostics, medical devices or vaccines. The report made recommendations to governments, international organisations, industry, civil society and other stakeholders addressing the relationship among IPR, access to health technologies, incentives for research and development and the opportunities to strengthen governance, accountability and transparency.

The principle recommendation of the panel was that World Trade Organization (WTO) members should commit themselves to respect at the highest political levels, the letter and spirit of Doha Declaration on TRIPS and Public Health refraining from any action that will limit its implementation and use in order to promote access to health technologies.

Some of the important recommendations in the report include:

➢ Governments must urgently increase their current levels of investment in health technology innovation to meet unmet needs and they should enter into negotiations for a binding research and development (R&D) treaty that delinks the costs of innovation from the end prices of health technologies in order to address issues that existing innovation mechanisms have failed to adequately address.

➢ There must be much greater transparency to ensure that the costs of research and development, production, marketing, and distribution, as well as the end prices of health technologies are clear to consumers and governments.

➢ Governments and the private sector must refrain from explicit or implicit threats, tactics or strategies that undermine the right of WTO members to use TRIPS flexibilities as reaffirmed in the Doha Declaration on TRIPS and Public Health. WTO members must register complaints against undue political and economic pressure and take punitive measures against offending members.

➢ The SG should establish an independent review body tasked with assessing progress on health technology innovation and access and for an HLM on Health Technology Innovation and Access to be convened by 2018.

The recommendations cover TRIPS flexibilities and TRIPS plus provisions, publicly funded research, new incentives for research and development of health technologies and governance and transparency issues in governments, private industry and multilateral organisations concerning R&D, production, pricing and distribution of health technologies, clinical trials and patent information.

The report of the panel became controversial with the United States and private industry, calling it biased. However, countries including India, Brazil and others pushed for the report to be discussed in forums including the WHO, WTO and the UN Human Rights Council. Attempts by member nations to push through a resolution in the World Health Assembly of WHO failed because of fragmentation in the coalition of developing countries who came together to push for greater and cheaper access to medicines. But high prices of drugs in international markets also brought unexpected support from some developed countries namely The Netherlands, Norway, Canada and Austria.

Over the next 1 year the recommendations of the HLP that had gained momentum with member states were those on transparency, including several proposals and strategies to increase transparency on pricing data, patent information, clinical trials and cost of R&D. In the World Health Assembly of May 2019 a draft resolution on Improving Transparency of Markets for Medicines, Vaccines and other health products proposed a broad range of interventions to improve global transparency on a variety of components relevant to health technology innovation and access including on clinical trial outcomes; prices; revenues; R&D costs; public sector investments and subsidies for R&D; marketing costs; patent and other related information. While the resolution was eventually adopted, much of its original content including provisions calling for increased transparency on R&D costs was watered down at the insistence of some member states.

The HLP report recommended 'The UNGA should convene a special session no later than 2018 on high technology innovation and access to agree on strategies and an accountability framework that will accelerate efforts towards promoting innovation and ensuring access as set out in the 2030 agenda'.

But because of the controversial nature of the recommendations with some high-income countries and the pharmaceutical industry opposing them, not much headway could be made until now to convene a special session of the UNGA on high technology innovation.

DEVELOPMENTS ON CRIMINAL LAW IN INDIA AND UGANDA

In the midst of all these developments, we had a huge setback on the legal front in India. On 11 December 2013, the Supreme Court of India overruled the 4-year old decision of the Delhi High Court, which had struck down India's anti-sodomy law, Section 377 of the Indian Penal Code (IPC). The path breaking judgement of Delhi High Court striking down the part of Section 377 IPC so far as it relates to consensual adult sex as ultra vires raised the aspirations of MSM and transgender community not just in India but in Asian and Caribbean countries which were former British colonies for a more friendly legal environment to emerge. But the Supreme Court's judgement disappointed many people around the world including the commissioners of the Global Commission on HIV and Law. We reacted with a statement conveying 'great dismay at this regressive step taken to dismantle a beacon of human rights articulation that was the Delhi High Court judgment'. We expressed our dismay that 'by suggesting that it is for Parliament to decide on retaining or removing Section 377, the Indian Supreme Court has articulated an atypical approach, removed from the great tradition of judicial review through public interest litigation developed by it over the past several decades and admired globally'. We joined the UNOHCHR in calling upon the Indian Supreme Court to review its decision and uphold the Delhi High Court verdict at the earliest so that more lives are not damaged by a moribund legislation in one of the flourishing democracies of the 21st century.

But it was not until another 4 years in 2018, a 5-judge constitutional bench of the SC consisting of chief justice and four other judges started hearing the challenge to constitutionality of Section 377. The Government of India did not take a position on the issue and left it to the 'wisdom of the court' to decide on Section 377. The petitioners invoked the right to sexual privacy, dignity, right against discrimination and freedom of expression to argue against the constitutionality of Section 377. After hearing the petitioners' plea the bench pronounced its verdict on 6 September 2018, reversing its own 2013 judgement of restoring Section 377 by stating that using the section of the IPC to victimize homosexuals was unconstitutional, and henceforth, a criminal act. In its ruling, the SC stated that consensual sexual acts between adults cannot be a crime, deeming the prior law 'irrational, arbitrary and incomprehensible.'

The Commission took a similar stand with regard to the HIV Prevention and AIDS Control Act passed by the Ugandan Parliament on 13 May 2014. The act contained punitive provisions including the imposition of lengthy custodial sentences for the intentional transmission of HIV (up to 10 years) and attempted transmission (up to 5 years).

We wrote to the Ugandan Government 'The HIV Prevention and AIDS Control Act was enacted despite an overwhelming body of evidence cited in our report and several other sources which show the harmful impact of these well-intentioned but ultimately misguided laws. Sadly, these developments in Uganda are not isolated. Our report found that more than 60 countries around the world have criminalised at least one aspect of HIV transmission, exposure or non-disclosure. ..... Most of the progress we have seen in the AIDS response has been founded on laws, policies and practices that are based on scientific evidence and grounded in human rights. We call for the President of Uganda to reject this Act which poses a grave danger to the hard gotten gains of its AIDS response'.

The UNDP secretariat through their monthly newsletters was keeping everyone in the UN system updated on the progress of legal reforms based on the recommendations of the Commission. These informative updates were very useful to monitor on various fronts, positive and negative developments on the legal environment.

CONFLATION OF SEX WORK AND TRAFFICKING

In February 2013, I received a notice from Pradip Ghosh, Senior Advocate SC of India that the SC constituted an experts panel to examine the issue of 'Prevention of Trafficking and Sex work'. He asked me to attend a day-long consultative meeting and share my experiences and perspective. The Global Commission on HIV and Law had a detailed examination of the issue and the possible conflation of sex work and trafficking in legislations enacted by national governments.

In my presentation to the panel I spoke about the Global Commission recommendations on sex work and anti-trafficking that,

'The Commission fully recognised the need to ensure criminal sanctions against human trafficking for purposes of commercial sexual exploitation and the careful use of such sanctions targeted to punish those using force to procure people into commercial sex......

International anti-human-trafficking campaigns often promote the prohibition, either intentional or effective, of proven best practices in HIV prevention. For instance, crusaders in the United States have used the influence of PEPFAR—the President's Emergency Plan for AIDS Relief, the primary vehicle of United States financial support to AIDS-combating organisations around the world—to compel other governments to accept the conflation of human trafficking with sex work by conditioning the receipt of funds on the signing of its Anti-Prostitution Pledge......Countries must....ensure that the enforcement of anti-human-trafficking laws is carefully targeted to punish those who use force, dishonesty or coercion to procure people into commercial sex, or who abuse migrant sex workers through debt bondage, violence or by deprivation of liberty. Anti-human-trafficking laws must be used to prohibit sexual exploitation and they must not be used against adults involved in consensual sex work.'

In my intervention I pointed out that the current legal framework of Immoral Trafficking Prevention Act (ITPA) in India based on international normative standards was highly punitive, rightfully aimed at bringing traffickers to book. Yet, it was not necessarily yielding the desired results in curbing trafficking. Anti-trafficking law, in the manner of its framing and implementation, has the brutal effect of punishing individuals engaging in sex work–the lowest hanging fruit, as they were the most disempowered and therefore the easiest to oppress through the long arm of the law. Indeed 90% of those who have been arrested under ITPA were sex workers, instead of those who traffic others into sex work.

In the end I recommended that any attempt made by the government to criminalise clients should be discouraged. This will create more problems than solving and enhances the misery and stigma of sex workers. Evidence was there to show that the Swedish example on which this model was based had failed to deliver the results in Sweden itself.

India as the largest democracy of the world should set an example in upholding the rights of underprivileged and marginalised sections of population namely sex workers and sexual minorities. Justice A.P. Shah in his landmark judgement striking off Section 377 of IPC criminalising same-sex relations had observed that tolerance and inclusiveness are part of our culture which should be preserved. Sex workers also deserve such inclusive policies which address stigma and discrimination practised by mainstream society.

I followed it up with an article in *Hindustan Times* headed 'Separating consent from exploitation.'[3]

ADVOCACY MISSIONS TO PRIORITY COUNTRIES

The UNAIDS secretariat in Geneva provided support to the Special Envoys by organising regular briefings and coordinating our advocacy visits to the countries. The UN resident coordinator system was informed about our missions to prepare local visits and meetings with senior political leaders and policy makers. We were periodically invited to UN headquarters to meet the UNSG Ban Ki-moon to update him on our work and set priorities. He always attached great importance to the work of the Special Envoys on AIDS and was especially sensitive to the problems of key populations and the stigma they encountered. Next 5 years was an exciting period of work which gave us a rare insight into the global level politics impacting on AIDS response and how they alternated between high-level optimism and deep despair.

I was quite familiar with the country-level AIDS responses in Asia Pacific region because of my work as RST Director in Bangkok. I kept some key countries on priority for advocacy and monitoring as the SE of UNSG instead of spreading my efforts too thin. Countries with high disease burden such as India, China, Thailand, Cambodia, Indonesia, Myanmar and Vietnam accounted for almost 90% of the disease burden in the region and were on my priority list. Small but key countries such as Nepal and Philippines also needed attention. China was getting directly monitored by Geneva with the EXD UNAIDS making periodical visits to pursue China–Africa partnership for getting assistance for AIDS programmes in African countries. I did not want a monitoring overload to happen in China and kept it out of my list.

INDIA'S AIDS RESPONSE

After a 5-year gap I got an opportunity to look at India's AIDS response from close quarters. The third phase of national programme (NACP III) as a vastly scaled-up response in India succeeded in bringing down new infections rates to 50% of 2001 level in 10 years. Antiretroviral therapy (ART) coverage had increased to 315,000 in 2010. Still there was overall concern about slowing down of the response amidst a spate of governance reforms starting from 2009. In that year, the government decided upon creation of a separate department of AIDS control (DAC) for the national AIDS programme and upgraded the position of director general (NACO) to a full-fledged secretary to government. The incumbent DG, Sujatha Rao, was promoted as Secretary of the Department. In the process DAC became a department with a single national programme for prevention and control of AIDS and administering NACP III. NACO still existed and was reporting to DAC, but the existence of two units, NACO and DAC, and their relationship was not clearly understood by the communities and people at large. One offshoot was that the financial control that existed in government departments with the presence of a senior official looking after internal financial control now got extended to DAC also. This had robbed the financial autonomy NACO enjoyed with delegated administrative and financial powers since it was established in 1992.

When the secretary Sujatha Rao ultimately left DAC in October 2009 to become the Health Secretary, I expected that government will restore NACO to its previous status and keep the strong link with Department of Health under the ministry. But that didn't happen and the department continued its existence. There was a quick succession of secretaries in DAC with four of them rotating in a period of 5 years (2008–2013). For every one of them DAC was not a position they wished to continue for long as it was a small unit compared to the Health and other larger departments in government. Later evidence had shown that the quick turnover of senior officials heading the national AIDS response adversely impacted the NACP IV, which was launched in 2012.

Another change which baffled civil society partners was the sudden change of incumbent in the key position of Joint Director Information Education and Communication (IEC) in NACO. This position which needed a strong civil society linkage was managed by officers from the Indian Information Service (IIS), a central civil service specialising in mass communications and interaction with media. Since the time I headed NACO, senior IIS officials–Neelam Kapur, Sadhana Rout and Mayank Agarwal provided the vital civil society link to the national programme and actively promoted mass communication and school education programmes. They were eminently suited to hold these positions because of their exposure to civil society organisations (CSOs) and non-health functionaries in other wings of government. It was not clear why DAC had chosen to revert such a functionary and opted to allot the work to Central Health Service officials who were medical doctors and not exposed to CSO work.

I believe that with these two changes in the governance structure civil society started losing its strategic link with the national programme with DAC acquiring more of a bureaucratic image.

During this period there was considerable anxiety with regard to the stand taken by the Planning Commission, the policy making body of government that all health programmes including NACP should be mainstreamed and administered through the newly created National Health Mission (NHM). The NHM, created in 2005/06 was settling down and already had an overload of national programmes for control of malaria, tuberculosis (TB), leprosy added to its charge. It would have been a disastrous step if NACP with a strong community link was mainstreamed midway through the national response. I joined a group of civil society and community representatives who got together as a civil society forum and met the Member for Health, Sayeda Ahmed, in Planning Commission to make a strong representation against merger of NACP with NHM. We were all relieved that the Government of India finally decided against the merger and kept NACP as an independent programme under the DAC.

In 2014, after the National Democratic Alliance (NDA) government assumed office, the DAC was abolished as a part of minimum governance policy of the new government and NACO was restored to its original position under the health ministry. This move was widely criticised by civil society activists and the media as an attempt to wind up NACO and merge the programme with the NHM. However, I was personally happy with this development as NACO needed the support of the mainstream health department and the Directorate General of Health Services (DGHS) as it was functionally not viable as an independent department.

I decided to include a mission to India as SESG to make a quick assessment of the state of response and the administrative changes brought about in the past few years. I and Steve Kraus, the RST Director, led a joint mission to India in February 2015 and met the new Health Secretary, Bhanu Pratap Sharma, the new Additional Secretary Navreet Kang in charge of NACO, the Mission Director of NHM and other senior functionaries and community representatives. We made a field visit to Punjab and met the state government officials implementing the programme. In the aide memoire we sent to the government after our visit, we requested the government to reestablish the position of DG NACO with all delegated financial and administrative powers and restore the cut in NACO budget to ensure full-scale implementation of NACP IV. We requested for a revamp of the National AIDS Committee (NAC) which hadn't met for a long time to make it small and compact and to have regular meetings for monitoring the national response. (*Aide memoire to Government of India, 23 February 2015.*)

I was happy to see that government designated Navreet Kang as DG NACO with all administrative and financial powers restored under the 1992 delegation order. But there was no follow-up on the other important suggestions we made. Kang who earlier worked in NACO had promptly tried to restore the ties with CSOs and community representatives and there was considerable optimism that the programme will once again receive the desired priority in the government.

PAKISTAN

There was concern about AIDS response in Pakistan, a country with 190 million people where new infections were on the rise contrary to the regional trend of overall decline. I visited Pakistan in 2005 as the Regional Director of UNAIDS and that was almost a decade ago. Marc Saba, the UCD in Pakistan invited me and Steve Kraus, the UNAIDS RST Director, to undertake an advocacy mission to engage the government for stronger efforts to control the epidemic. We visited Islamabad on a 3-day mission in April 2014 and met the new health minister, the minister for development and planning and senior programme officials and civil society partners. On the final day we had a meeting with the President of Pakistan and apprised him about our findings on the national AIDS response and recommendations. The security situation in the country did not enable us to travel outside Islamabad.

We realised that an important reason for the slowing down of AIDS response in Pakistan was the Constitutional Amendment in 2011 abolishing the Ministry of Health at the federal level. The intention of the amendment was to devolve more powers to the provinces which was a progressive move. But the country needed a nodal ministry to coordinate national efforts and for accountability at international level. The provinces got more money and resources but lacked the technical capacity that was critical to administer a programme such as HIV/AIDS. This was a unique situation which probably did not exist in any other country. The *Lancet* commented 'Pakistan could be the first country without an institutional structure—a ministry, state department, directorate, or equivalent structure—at the federal level in charge of national responsibilities for health'.

Lancet went on to add,
'This amendment comes at a time when there is a dire need to increase the capacity of the health system in view of many serious challenges......
There are many national responsibilities for health in federal systems, including health information, regulation, international commitments, trade in health, establishment of policy norms and standards, and

interprovincial policy coordination. These responsibilities have to be centrally managed.'[4]

In May 2013, the new government reinstated the federal ministry for heath naming it as the Ministry of National Health Services, Regulation and Coordination. The national programmes for control of AIDS and TB were kept under the charge of the federal ministry while many other health programmes were devolved to the provincial governments. But in the intervening 2 years the provincial governments assumed full authority and were very reluctant to get back to the earlier system of remaining accountable to the federal government. This change in governance structures had a deep impact on the AIDS programme and the country lost an opportunity to bring the epidemic under control.

By the time we visited Pakistan the federal ministry was trying to reestablish its mandate under the new Health Minister Saira Afzal Tarar who explained to us the transition problems she was experiencing in bringing the provinces on a common accountability framework. In the aide memoire we left with the government at the end of the visit, we highlighted the problems such as lack of political will, sub-optimal financing and absence of required scale-up of prevention and treatment programmes which were hindering progress and failing to make an impact on the spread of the epidemic in the country. The epidemic which was initially confined to 12 cities in Pakistan was now spreading to the rural areas also. We welcomed the devolution to the provinces but wanted strategic information, monitoring and evaluation and provision of required level of funding to stay as core responsibilities of the federal government.

MYANMAR

In October 2014, I had to visit Myanmar to attend a civil society dialogue called Blue Sky Week organised by the International HIV/AIDS Alliance, an international NGO registered in United Kingdom. I joined the alliance as a board member in 2010. I was planning to do a country mission to Myanmar for some time and thought this would be a good opportunity to combine both the events. Eamonn Murphy, the new UNAIDS Country Director, welcomed this plan and arranged the country mission at a very short notice.

After attending the programmes of the Blue Sky Week in Yangon, I travelled to Nay Pyi Taw, the Myanmar capital with Eamonn where we met senior political leaders including the health minister, minister in president's office, the deputy ministers of foreign affairs and home and the attorney general. We also met Daw Suu Kyi, the leader of opposition and a popular woman leader in Asia. Back in Yangon, we attended a meeting organised by the UCO with the civil society representatives on the post-2015 development agenda. The general elections in late 2015 were awaited with great expectations as an important determinant in the march of the country towards a fully democratic system of governance.

Myanmar was not sufficiently engaged in the post-2015 development process, and during my meetings I kept this issue as priority. I requested the top political leadership to proactively get engaged in the post-2015 development agenda and to support 'ending AIDS' as an important goal within the SDG on health. I got very positive response from them and the Deputy Minister of Foreign Affairs wanted us to organise a briefing session for his diplomats on this matter.

I also raised the issue of legal reforms in Myanmar which were needed to improve access to prevention and treatment services to vulnerable populations. The Ministry of Home Affairs agreed to reissue the instructions not to use condoms as evidence to arrest key population groups in its effort to encourage cooperation between the health and law enforcement sectors.

The ministry was also planning to amend the 1993 Narcotic Law to make treatment voluntary and expand access. I recommended that the registration of drug users may be dispensed with in keeping with the recommendations of the Global Commission on HIV and Law. For this purpose, I extended help from UNAIDS to facilitate consultation with key partners and civil society on the draft amendment.

I also alerted them to the possibility of scaled down funding from international donors including Global Fund when Myanmar graduates into a middle-income country. I and Eamonn offered to support them to work out a financial transition plan to project the requirement and availability of domestic and foreign resources for AIDS programmes for the next 10 years.

The health minister welcomed the offer. (*Aide Memoire–SESG's Myanmar visit, 17 October 2014.*)

Myanmar, despite the prevailing political uncertainty and limited external funding, had managed to keep the HIV infections levels under control. Civil society had always been very active in prevention programmes for drug user and sex worker communities. Above all, the government managed to keep efficient and technically sound programme managers at leadership level in the national response.

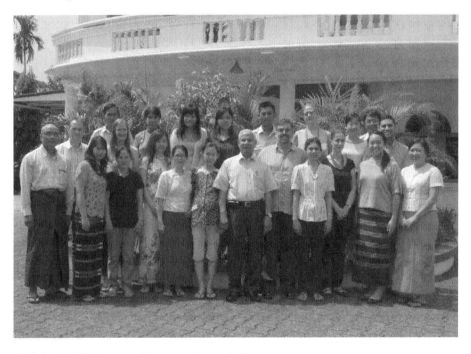

With the UNAIDS Country Director and team in Myanmar

INDONESIA

Two key countries which were witnessing the same challenge of the epidemic breaking free after relative periods of stability were Indonesia and Philippines.

Kah Sin Cho who worked in my team as Regional Programme Advisor in RST Bangkok was positioned as the new country director of UNAIDS in Indonesia. We discussed the Indonesian situation and decided that

I should do an advocacy mission in this third most populous country in Asia. During my mission to Indonesia in October 2015, we noticed that compared to the spirited response to AIDS we witnessed in 2008 under the leadership of Nafsiah M'boi as Secretary of NAC, there were clear signs of slowing down of programme implementation mainly at the provincial level without any effective check from the federal government. I was concerned at the organised attempt by government to wipe out sex worker colonies through raids and detention. The minister in charge of Women Empowerment whom I met during the mission proudly declared that she had already demolished 122 out of 136 prostitution sites and was on course to achieve her target of 'elimination' of brothels in Indonesia by 2019! Sex workers, drug users and other key populations were not getting required access to prevention and treatment services, which was the main reason for increasing rate of new infections.

There were some bright spots such as the Governor of Jakarta, Basuki Tjahaja Purnama, providing support to communities of sex workers and MSM for testing and ARV treatment. He promised all support to the UNAIDS initiative 'Fast Track Cities' for focused programming in all mega cities in the world.

At the end of the visit I tried to impress in my aide memoire that low coverage of prevention and treatment interventions and conflicting laws between the national and provincial governments were the main inhibiting factors to a full-scale response to AIDS in the country.

I stressed, 'In a country such as Indonesia with a decentralised administrative set up, the sub-national governments play a key role in shaping the local laws and regulation for development. However, there are many conflicting laws and regulations that impede the effective response to AIDS. I am especially concerned that national program on HIV prevention in sexual transmission is being undermined by the closure of brothel complexes across the country. I am concerned that the harm reduction program is being undermined by a punitive approach to drug use'. (*Aide memoire to Government of Indonesia, 29 October 2015.*)

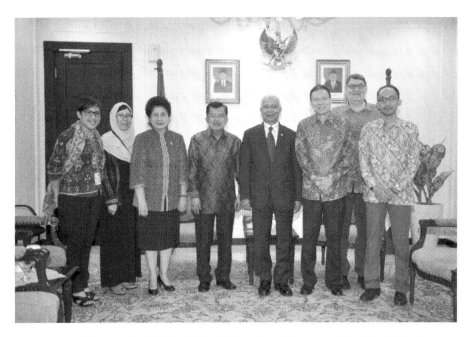

With Vice President Yusuf Kalla (fourth from left) and Health Minister (third from left) of Indonesia

PHILIPPINES

The Philippines story was even more tragic. During my mission in August 2013, I was alarmed to see that after lying dormant for many years the HIV epidemic had really grown in size and prevalence in the past 3 years. 'The prevalence levels among key populations at risk, particularly men who have sex with men, injecting drug users, and freelance sex workers have increased manifold. The overall low prevalence among general population masks this rising trend and gives an impression that the situation is under control. It is therefore a challenge for the programme implementors to sensitize leaders and people at large to make them understand the true nature of this looming epidemic'. (*Aide memoire Philippines Mission, 30 August 2013.*)

In the past few years after my mission, situation only got worse. There was an outbreak of HIV among 136 prison inmates in Cebu who were all drug users, apparently due to sharing of infected needles. The declaration of a 'war on drugs' by President Duterte and the extra judicial killings of young drug users put the entire prevention programme for drug users on the back burner. There was ample testimony from number of reports, that such a policy will not work–the latest from the report of the Global Commission on HIV and Law. But no one could have put it more forcefully than a former President of Colombia who learnt from his experience that such a policy will fail in the long run. In an OpEd in *New York Times* he said,

'While the Filipino government has a duty to provide for the security of its people, there is a real risk that a heavy-handed approach will do more harm than good. There is no doubt that tough penalties are necessary to deter organized crime. But extrajudicial killings and vigilantism are the wrong ways to go. After the killing of a South Korean businessman, Mr. Duterte seemed as if he might be closer to realizing this. But bringing the army in to fight the drug war, as he now suggests, would also be disastrous. The fight against drugs has to be balanced so that it does not infringe on the rights and well-being of citizens.......... Taking a hard line against criminals is always popular for politicians. I was also seduced into taking a tough stance on drugs during my time as President. The polls suggest that Mr. Duterte's war on drugs is equally popular. But he will find that it is unwinnable. I also discovered that the human costs were enormous. We could not win the war on drugs through killing petty criminals and addicts. We started making positive impacts only when we changed tack, designating drugs as a social problem and not a military one'.[5]

I was disturbed to see the sharp decline in coverage of key populations with focused prevention programmes in priority countries which contribute to a large disease burden. In an internal communication to UNAIDS Headquarters I recorded my impression after my Indonesia mission.

'It is established beyond doubt by evidence that the key to reduction of new infections and thus seeing the end of AIDS lies in saturating prevention and treatment services to key populations (KPs). It is ironical that these very programs are not getting enough mileage with Governments. In fact we are seeing a reversal of gains with KPs getting more and more criminalised with a plethora of local laws getting enacted totally contradictory to national legislations. Indonesia is a classic example. And all this is happening in the name of decentralisation.

It is good to be optimistic about ending AIDS but it is also time that we stop being euphoric about it as it is hurting civil society sentiment. There are enormous challenges with AIDS control losing momentum and being 'passed on' to provinces and local bodies without any lines of accountability established for performance and for following national policies and guidelines.

I feel we should do some tough talking without trying to be unduly diplomatic in the run up to HLM 2016.We must face the political leadership with hard questioning and should not mince words that after a period of relative success in halting the epidemic, they are slipping back into complacency. And the cases of four Asian countries, Indonesia, Pakistan, Philippines and Malaysia (I did't know the actual situation in China) which are seeing increasing rates of infections year after year, are all the more serious'.

And I received a candid reply.

'It is clear that we need to have a very serious discussion in-house to figure out if and when to use this phrase, (ending AIDS) its risks and benefits, and perhaps most important, its meaning! I very much hope we will have a clear message along the following lines; We have the biomedical tools that in theory allow us to end AIDS. But ending AIDS will be very difficult. It requires greater resources for prevention and treatment, sustained commitment over the next few generations and perhaps most challenging- reaching highly marginalized and criminalized populations at a scale we are nowhere near. This last will require a different level of political commitment, different ways of outreach and a great deal of human rights work to overcome political, legal and social barriers'.

CAMBODIA

In the midst of this disappointing scenario, one beacon of hope was Cambodia, a country which made enormous progress on the AIDS front since the 1990s. By 2014, numbers of new infections were brought down from a high of 8821 in 2001 to a mere 692 and the overall prevalence rate to 0.7% from a high of 1.8% in 2001. About 78% of those eligible were covered with ART and despite its limited resource mobilisation capability the government was able to allocate sufficient resources for AIDS programmes. Mortality due to AIDS was brought down from a high of over 10,000 in 2003 to 2700 in 2015. With a strong political commitment and resource back up, Cambodia was the only Asian country to reach the 2015 targets on prevention and treatment set under the 2011 Political Declaration adopted in the HLM on AIDS at UNGA.

NEPAL

In my last mission as SE to UNSG, Steve and I visited Nepal in September 2016. We had meetings with the Health Minister Gagan Thapa, Deputy Prime Minister and Minister of Home Affairs, Bimalendra Nidhi, Deputy Prime Minister and Minister of Finance Krishna Bahadur Mahara and several senior officials in the Ministry of Health and the National Center for AIDS and STD Control. We rounded up our mission with a meeting with the Vice Chair of the National Planning Board, Bahadur Shresta. We also met with civil society networks and community groups to understand the impact of rapidly changing political scenario on national AIDS responses. During our interactions with the government functionaries we tried to obtain responses on: What it takes in terms of smart investments to achieve the fast-track targets? How does the government want to secure these resources? What are the mechanisms of fund flows to implementing agencies; both government and nongovernment and what are the bottlenecks?

Nepal's record in AIDS response was always commendable in the background of severe resource constraints and constantly changing political environment. It was estimated that 39,000 people were living with HIV in Nepal, at the end of 2015. The country recorded a significant decline in new infections down from 7400 in 2001 to 1300 in 2015; a drop of 82%. However, treatment coverage was only 30% with 12,000 people getting ART. Nepal had to depend largely on external assistance for its AIDS programme. Currently, about US $18 million were being invested in Nepal's HIV response, with only about 15% from domestic resources. To fast track the HIV response by 2020, it was estimated that annually US $ 30 to 40 million will be required over the next 5 years.

In a detailed aide memoir submitted at the conclusion of the mission we emphasised that in order to achieve the fast-track target of reducing new infections, Nepal should have no more than 500 new infections by 2020; a reduction of 90% over the 2010 level.

To achieve this target, strategic investment on nondiscriminatory coverage of key populations needed to be scaled-up and intensified. A test and treat policy, if adopted, will help in covering more than 22,000 adults and children with ART to achieve the fast-track targets.

The new government favourably responded to the recommendations and asked for technical help from UNAIDS and financial support from GFATM as a least developed country.

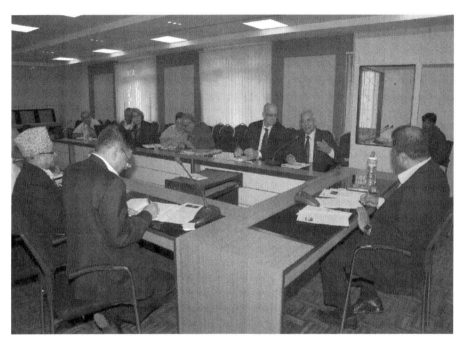

Meeting with the Vice Chair of the National Planning Board, Nepal, along with Steve Kraus and Ruben del Prado, UNAIDS country director

In all my country missions I got tremendous support from the resident coordinators and other country directors of the UN system which demonstrated the multi-sectoral nature of the joint UN programme on AIDS. Steve, his successor Eamonn and the country directors of UNAIDS in the priority countries attached great importance to the country missions and tried to do an effective follow-up on the recommendations presented to the governments at the end of the missions.

HIGH-LEVEL PANEL ON AIDS FUNDING LANDSCAPE FOR ASIA PACIFIC

As the countries were gearing up their efforts towards the run up to the post-2015 development agenda, UNAIDS and the World Bank came together in August 2013 to make an objective evaluation of the AIDS funding scenario in Asia Pacific by an independent panel of experts. The agencies felt that Asia Pacific region will face a serious funding challenge for AIDS programmes as more and more countries in the region graduate to middle-income level resulting in fast drying up of external funding. Due to global economic recession several large donor countries adopted austerity measures and shifted their funding priorities. Without assured scale-up of funding from both domestic and external resources, all the gains of the past decade could get wiped out. The panel was tasked to look at various funding options and probable scenarios for the progression of the epidemic and response. I was asked to chair the panel which consisted of 11 members drawn from countries, independent experts and civil society representatives. The Kirby Institute in New South Wales, Australia, was selected to do modelling studies for making projections on funding scenarios for 2020. The RST UNAIDS with Marlyn Borromeo, the regional programme advisor as point person, provided secretarial and funding support for the panel's work.

It was an exciting work for me as it addressed a very critical area of funding for fast-tracking AIDS programmes in the next 7 to 8 years. We had some teething problems with the research findings from Kirby Institute, but could iron them with a team of external technical experts reviewing the projections. The panel felt that a unidirectional approach in projecting the future will leave the country's leadership with a yes or no option only. Instead a scenarios' approach was adopted with various options to enable the countries to take informed decisions on investing resources for AIDS programmes.

After making an interim presentation on the findings and possible recommendations in the International AIDS Conference in Melbourne in 2014, the panel finally came out with its Report 'Investing in Results–how Asia Pacific countries can invest for ending AIDS' containing nine broad recommendations for charting a new course forward. These were based on five likely scenarios for AIDS treatment and prevention funding until 2020. We took a considered decision not to go beyond 2020 in view of the fast-changing economic environment in the region. The scenarios ranged from a business as usual approach to significant expansion of HIV prevention and treatment programmes. The recommendations focused on a set of rapid and carefully considered adjustments that would reach 80% of key populations with effective prevention services and provide testing and treatment services to at least 80% of people living with HIV by 2020.

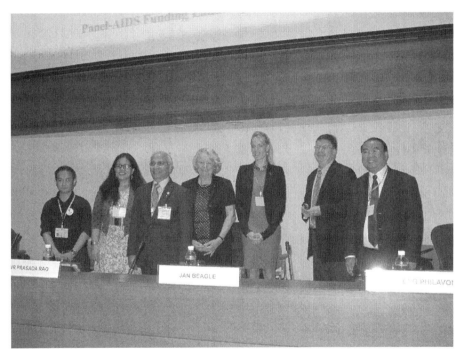

Presenting the report at the International AIDS Conference in Melbourne 2014

In the best-case scenario the region would see a steep drop in annual new infections to about 192,000 by 2020 and AIDS-related deaths would decrease to about 98,000. In a worst-case scenario where prevention coverages actually diminish and treatment remains at current coverage, the annual new infections would increase to about 391,000 in 2020 and keep growing at a quick pace. AIDS-related deaths would hover around 400,000 and keep increasing.

We recommended introducing funding transition plans supported by bridge funding options for middle-income countries and asked them to develop 'investment cases' for designing and costing high impact, rights-based and sustainable AIDS responses. Already some countries were in the process of developing investment cases which could be technically supported by UN agencies. The panel recommended that countries should invest resources in programmes producing maximum impact–reiterating the earlier stand taken by the Commission on AIDS in Asia in 2008. Developing new financial streams by introducing a tax or levy to finance a health promotion fund with a portion earmarked for AIDS programmes was another important recommendation of the panel. For treatment programmes the panel asked countries to follow the WHO treatment guidelines and use the simplest drug regimens, the most effective treatment support methods and economical administrative systems. The panel observed that some countries were purchasing an unnecessarily wide range of ARV drugs leading to inefficiencies in the supply chain.

We expressed the hope that Asia Pacific region could become the first region to end AIDS as a public threat by 2030 if it makes the right strategic choices using its ability to mobilise additional resources, a vibrant civil society and the capacity to manufacture and supply affordable generic drugs for treatment.

The report of the panel which was another trendsetter for the region was released at the high-profile Asia Pacific Intergovernmental meeting on HIV/AIDS organised by UNESCAP in January 2015.

The latest epidemic profile of HIV provides an interesting comparison with the projections made by the panel for 2020. The number of new infections as per the latest estimates of UNAIDS stand at 300,000 for the region, a 100,000 more than the best case scenario predicted by the panel. The number of AIDS deaths reported at 160,000–almost double the number of the best case scenario. The numbers were not as high as in the worst case scenario either.

The conclusions are obvious. The region has not performed to its capacity in reducing new infections and AIDS-related mortality and would be missing the 2020 targets in the process!

SDGS AND POST-2015 DEVELOPMENT AGENDA

My appointment as SESG in 2012 coincided with a global mobilisation of public opinion towards sustainable development in the post-2015 era. The MDGs with a set of targets for achievement by 2015 had triggered unprecedented political activity to tackle the many dimensions of poverty. Though the performance of countries was mixed in achieving them, the MDGs met with several successes at country level.

The United Nations Conference on Sustainable Development in Rio de Janeiro from 20 to 22 June 2012 unleashed the agenda for sustainable development where the heads of governments with full participation of civil society renewed their commitment to sustainable development and to ensuring the promotion of an economically, socially and environmentally sustainable future for the planet and for present and future generations. The conference established an intergovernmental process that was open to all stakeholders to develop global SDGs to be agreed by the UNGA. An open working group (OWG) was constituted with 30 representatives nominated by member states from the 5 UN regional groups to define a new global agenda and submit its report to UNGA during the 68th session in 2014.

The conference report in its 283 articles defined the entire stretch of development agenda which included health and population as one of the thematic areas identified under the framework for action and follow-up. On communicable diseases the report emphasised 'the countries …..that HIV and AIDS, malaria, tuberculosis, influenza, polio and other communicable diseases remain serious global concerns, and committed to redouble efforts to achieve universal access to HIV prevention, treatment, care and support and to eliminate mother-to-child transmission of HIV, as well as to renew and strengthen the fight against malaria, tuberculosis and neglected tropical diseases'. (*Rio Declaration, 2012*)

The SG in pursuance of resolution adopted by the General Assembly (GA) on 22 September 2010, 'Keeping the promise: united to achieve the

Millennium Development Goals' submitted a report in 2013 outlining his vision for a post-2015 development agenda apart from reporting on the annual progress of MDGs. The SG's report made a strong pitch for poverty eradication as indispensable for sustainable development. On the specific issue of HIV/AIDS the SG reported the impressive progress in the last decade 'New HIV infections declined by 21 per cent globally over the past decade, and close to 10 million people living with HIV are receiving lifesaving antiretroviral treatment. Expanded treatment and prevention yielded a 25 per cent reduction in AIDS-related deaths between 2005 and 2011. Yet 2.5 million new infections still occur each year and in many parts of the globe, millions lack access to treatment'.[6]

In his first meeting with us in January 2013, SG Ban Ki-moon identified post-2015 development agenda as one of the focus areas for the SEs to help him communicate his vision on global health development and social security. Substantial part of my work time as SE for the next 2 years was therefore devoted to events connected with the post-2015 development agenda. The SG appointed a new High Level Panel (HLP) of eminent persons in July 2012 to make recommendations on the post-2015 development agenda with three cochairs, the President of Indonesia, the President of Liberia and the Prime Minister of United Kingdom. He wanted us to participate in related meetings of the panel and give our inputs on AIDS programmes.

An important regional event contributing to this agenda was the Asian parliamentarians' call for sustained action to end AIDS. The call came at a forum held at Bali, Indonesia, on 25 and 26 March 2013, where parliamentarians and civil society leaders from 35 countries in the Asia Pacific region came together to critically assess achievements and challenges of the MDGs in the region and to suggest a common roadmap to the HLP of eminent persons. I attended the meeting along with Steve Kraus and provided inputs to the Bali declaration issued at the end of the meeting. In the declaration the forum called for sustained action on AIDS towards ensuring an AIDS-free generation–carrying forward the MDG agenda beyond 2015. My appeal as SESG was to carry the MDG agenda beyond 2015 with an emphasis on equity and ensuring services for the most marginalised in our societies. I recommended an overarching post-2015 goal built around the 'healthy planet for healthy people' premise and an increase in public expenditure on health to at least 3% of gross domestic product (GDP) to enable universal access to health and attainment of health goals.

'With political commitment, community mobilization, adequate funding and the right approaches, the end of AIDS and the emergence of an AIDS-free generation can be a shared triumph of the post-2015 era', I said during my intervention.

The report of the HLP submitted in May 2013, offered a powerful vision that builds on the MDGs and proposed to address unfinished business from the MDGs and offered a path towards prosperity and the fulfillment of human rights and dignity.

The panel recommended 12 universal goals. The panel observed that the benefits of investing in health outweigh costs 1 to 12 in preventing HIV/AIDS. But surprisingly the goal 'Ensuring Healthy Lives' contained a sub-goal 4e which stopped with the objective to 'reduce the burden of disease from HIV/AIDS tuberculosis, malaria, neglected tropical diseases and priority non communicable diseases'.

The panel's vaguely suggested target of reducing the burden of disease from HIV/AIDS came as a disappointment for many of us as it was not forceful enough to guide the countries towards elimination of AIDS as a public health threat. The MDG target of halting and reversing the epidemic by 2015 was much more emphatic. Along with UNAIDS we decided to continue with our advocacy with member countries of the OWG to recommend a more forceful target on AIDS like ending the epidemic as a public health threat by 2030.

UNAIDS as the joint UN programme launched into the preparatory action for defining the post-2015 agenda for AIDS, which was a historic opportunity to refocus country-level efforts towards the goals set in the declaration. A series of calls for ending AIDS originated from different quarters around the same time.

The African Union had called for ending AIDS, tuberculosis and malaria by 2030 and the United States Government for an AIDS-free generation.

The Washington DC Declaration, signed by thousands of organisations, public figures, advocates, scientists and practitioners worldwide, called for leadership and commitment to seize the opportunity of beginning to end the epidemic.

These advocacy efforts paid off and the report of the UNSG submitted to the GA in July 2013 was much more impactful and called for a future free of AIDS. On the health agenda for 2030, he called for universal health care coverage, access and affordability; ending preventable maternal and child deaths; realizing women's reproductive health and rights; increasing immunisation coverage; eradicating malaria and realising the vision of a future free of AIDS and TB; reducing the burden of noncommunicable diseases, including mental illness and road accidents and promoting healthy behaviours including those related to water, sanitation and hygiene.[7]

UNAIDS *LANCET* COMMISSION

As a parallel effort to focus global attention on accelerated AIDS response, the PCB of UNAIDS announced in 2012 that a new Commission will be jointly launched with Richards Horton of *Lancet* on 'AIDS to sustainable health'. The Commission was jointly chaired by President Joyce Banda of Malawi, Nkosazana Zuma, Chairman of the African Union Commission and Peter Piot, the then Director of Imperial College, London, with 17 other members. Drawing from the experience of global AIDS response, the Commission will marshal global leadership, expertise and momentum to shape the debate of future of health and accelerate the end of AIDS. The number of commissioners was increased to 31 by the time the first meeting was held. The SEs of UNSG were included as special invitees to the Commission meetings.

In the first meeting of the Commission held at Lilongwe, Malawi, in June 2013, three expert advisory panels were convened around each of the organising questions: (1) what will it take to end AIDS, (2) how can AIDS act as a pathfinder for health and development and (3) how to reform the AIDS governance architecture. The three panels were mandated to produce rigorous working papers in advance of the first Commission meeting as a core resource for the Commission in developing its recommendations. I attended the first Commission along with my fellow envoys from EECA and Caribbean regions.

In the Malawi meeting, Peter took a principled stand that HIV was not over and won't be over that easily and that fast. He cautioned that we should not fall for the myth of a silver bullet as no vaccine was going to be available anytime soon. I joined Helen Clark, Administrator UNDP to share our disappointment with the report of the HLPEP which did not contain a strong target for AIDS elimination as anticipated. I reminded the participants that AIDS will not be over without a determined effort. The slogan of ending AIDS should not make us euphoric that it was just round the corner. There was clear evidence of complacency at national level and prevention efforts were not getting implemented to scale. I strongly advocated that the Commission should advance alternative delivery models–shifting from government to the community ownership. I stressed the importance of commissioners finding ways to influence the intergovernmental processes leading to the negotiation of the post-2015 development agenda. I laid out a series of potential entry points for commissioners to influence the debate, both as individuals and as a Commission.

After an engaging 2 days the Commission's mandate was changed to 'defeating AIDS and advancing global health' which was considered more impactful in its message.

I was asked to play a more proactive role by joining the first working group and contribute to the debate on what would it take to end AIDS.

Working group 1 held its meeting through video conferences and concluded that

➢ Ending AIDS is possible and desirable and is imperative to the post-2015 agenda.

➢ End of AIDS will depend on building on successes, learning from failures and implementing to scale. This applies to both biomedical and social/structural interventions.

➢ AIDS will not end tomorrow but it has to be a part of our long-term vision.

A clearer set of recommendations, however, emerged from the Asia Pacific regional consultation held in Bangkok on 19 November 2013.

1. The concept of an AIDS-free world or the campaign to end AIDS still remain as abstract ideas which need unpacking into concrete policies, strategies and programmes. While it was agreed that an AIDS-free society is achievable, the time frame in which it could be accomplished needs to be broken down with intermediate targets and programmes to achieve them.

2. The post-2015 development agenda that will be negotiated in the GA in 2014-2015 needs to lay strong emphasis on clearly measurable targets for HIV prevention, care and support and improving the legal environment to be achieved by 2030. Clearly it was not envisaged that we reach all the three zeroes by that time. We therefore need intermediate targets/goals for 2030 which should have global consensus.

3. While the days of AIDS exceptionalism were over, we can't err on the other extreme of total integration in the name of taking AIDS out of isolation. We need to pitch it strategically somewhere in between. Programmes which are biomedical, for example treatment and PMTCT, could be gradually integrated into health systems while those which were focused on key populations such as prevention, legal environment and human rights need to be dealt exceptionally with intense and meaningful participation of key affected populations.

These recommendations were realistic, down to earth and hold good now more than at any time in the past.

I attended the second and final meeting of the Commission held at London in February 2014 where it agreed on the approach and the content of the report. The report was rich in content and tried to grapple with contradictory stands on the thrust of the messages. The challenge before the Commission was how much it should align itself with the UN agenda of ending AIDS, while recognising the ground level reality of growing complacency and heightened stigma and discrimination against key populations.

The report contained seven key recommendations, leading with the urgent need to scale-up AIDS efforts by getting serious about HIV prevention and expanding access to treatment. Efficient mobilisation of more resources for HIV prevention, treatment and research, and transparent governance and accountability for HIV and health were the other important ones. The Commission highlighted the need to expedite changes in laws, policies and attitudes that violate the rights of vulnerable populations, and that hinder an effective AIDS response.

Peter Piot, one of the cochairs of the Commission cautioned 'We must face hard truths—if the current rate of new HIV infections continues, merely sustaining the major efforts we already have in place will not be enough to stop deaths from AIDS increasing within five years in many countries......Expanding sustainable access to treatment is essential, but we will not treat ourselves out of the AIDS epidemic'.

One of the sobering findings from the report was that sustaining current HIV treatment and prevention efforts would require up to 2% of GDP, and at least a third of total government health expenditure from 2014 to 2030 to fund HIV programmes in the most affected African countries. This was a tall order for countries struggling to spend even 1% of GDP as public expenditure on health.

The Commission's report was targeted for publication in *Lancet* in February 2015 but could not be done until June 2015, a clear 1 year after the OWG report was finalised. It was launched only in July 2015 by SG Ban Ki-moon a couple of months before the UN HLM on the SDGs. In the process the report lost the opportunity to inform and influence the member states who that would be negotiating the SDGs for agreement by September 2015.

The OWG of countries released its report in July 2014 containing the important SDG target of ending AIDS by 2030 and agreed by acclamation to submit it to the GA at its 68th session in August 2014 for consideration and appropriate action. The SDG 3 'Ensure healthy lives and promote well-being for all at all ages' was accompanied with specific targets one of them being 'ending the epidemics of AIDS, tuberculosis, malaria and neglected tropical diseases by 2030 and combating hepatitis, water-borne diseases and other communicable diseases as well defined targets'. The SDGs, built on the foundation laid by the MDGs, sought to complete the unfinished business of the MDGs and respond to new challenges.

25 September 2015 marked the start of the UN Sustainable Development Summit and saw the official adoption of the 2030 agenda. It was a historic moment for me and fellow envoys, Michel Kazatchkine and Eddie Greene, to be present in the GA Hall to witness the adoption of the agenda. The outgoing and incoming presidents of the GA (former of Uganda, latter of Denmark), the UNSG and civil society representative spoke at the meeting.

Number of speakers filled the rest of the session including heads of state and government, UN organisations, civil society and the private sector. Prominent among them were President Obama from United States and Prime Minister Narendra Modi from India. Jan Beagle, Deputy EXD addressed the plenary on behalf of UNAIDS.

Our overall feeling was that the SDG Summit was a real triumph. In a fragmented and increasingly polarised world, it was quite remarkable that 136 heads of state and government and all 193 UN member states at some level of representation came together to adopt an agenda of unprecedented scope that recognised both the full extent of the major challenges of our day and that all countries and all sectors will be needed to respond to them.

The reception of the goals had undoubtedly been mixed–there were cynics who said that it was all a pipe dream and not precise enough to shift any agendas. But there were also those who were optimistic and recognised them as a great opportunity to change the world for the better. The message for civil society in coming years was well articulated by Transparency International, 'the SDGs offer an enormous opportunity to hold the feet of the world's leaders to the fire, to consistently and publicly remind them of their pledges and to demand actions on a scale and with an impact that builds a better world'.

For the UN family the SDGs offered a challenge which was very effectively conveyed by Helen Clark in her letter to UN Resident Coordinators and country teams which spoke to the need for change within the UN system: 'Transforming our world is a tall order. To be an integral part of this next fifteen year chapter of development history, we also have to transform ourselves'. For the joint UN programme on AIDS, the SDGs were a real opportunity to work together to make the transformative shifts to get the countries on track to ending AIDS by 2030 and to achieve all the SDGs.

But my excitement was short-lived with two important UN high-level meetings held in 2016–on Drugs and AIDS within a gap of 3 months showing that the old prejudices and attitudes towards vulnerable populations continue to persist in many countries and run counter to the unanimous support given by these very countries to the adoption of the SDGs at the UNGA in September 2015.

UNITED NATIONS GENERAL ASSEMBLY SPECIAL SESSION (UNGASS) ON DRUGS

In early April 2016, I and my wife took a short vacation in United States to visit my children and that greatly facilitated my participation in these two global events (1) the UNGASS on drugs in April 2016 and the HLM on AIDS in June 2016, with minimum expenditure to UNAIDS and ease of travel.

The UNGASS on drugs, convened from 19 to 21 April 2016, was meant to be an important milestone in achieving the goals set in the policy document of 2009, 'Political Declaration and Plan of Action on International Cooperation towards an Integrated and Balanced Strategy to Counter the World Drug Problem', which defined action to be taken by member states as well as goals to be achieved by 2019.

In preparation for the special session, the Commission on Narcotic Drugs (CND), the United Nations organisation with the prime responsibility for drug control matters, adopted in its 58th session a resolution entitled 'Special Session of the General Assembly on the World Drug Problem to be held in 2016', making recommendations on organisational and substantive matters regarding the session for adoption by the GA. The outcome document entitled, 'Our joint commitment to effectively addressing and countering the world drug problem' was transmitted to the GA recommending its adoption at the plenary of the UNGASS on the world drug problem.

Ahead of the UNGASS on drugs, UNAIDS released a strong and substantive report, 'Do No Harm; Health, Human Rights and People Who Use Drugs'. This report was warmly welcomed by many. But we were all surprised when the outcome document,' recommended by the CND was adopted as a resolution by the GA on 19 April 2016, on the first day of the session itself without any debate. The resolution, adopted without any discussion, had left the rest of the session for speeches by the country delegates supporting the resolution and relegating the large civil society participants and drug user communities to the sidelines.

The UNGASS outcome document generated mixed reactions and UNAIDS' own press release recognised where progress has been made but equally identified the shortcomings (not least the failure to mention harm-reduction explicitly) and pointed out the lack of progress on the 2011 Political Declaration commitment of reducing up to 50% of HIV infections among people who inject drugs. 'The war on drugs became a war on people and, for HIV it was not working' the document said.

I found the outcome document had disappointed many, especially the drug user community and agencies working on harm reduction programmes. In a side event organised by UNDP on aligning drug control efforts with the 2030 Sustainable Development Agenda, I as a panelist expressed my disappointment at the outcome document and absence of harm reduction as a policy and said,

'The outcome document is silent on some important priorities which are so critical to advance the cause of human development. It is silent on harm reduction as a policy and only speaks indirectly about needle syringe and oral substitution programmes, even though harm reduction has been widely endorsed and agreed, most prominently in the 2001 and 2011 Political Declarations on HIV/AIDS. Capital punishment is another controversial issue which does not find any mention in the document.

It still applauds the three international drug control conventions as the corner stone of international drug control system while successive Global Commissions on drugs and law have advocated for a revisit of these conventions as they have fallen short in making a difference to the world drug problem.

But if people, particularly the poor and most marginalised are to be the focus, and if alignment with the SDGs has to be the underlying theme of UNGASS 2016, we need to do much more. Drug policy cuts across core areas of sustainable development: health and well-being, gender equality, peace, justice and strong institutions amongst others. There has been growing attention to the harmful consequences of many drug control laws, policies and enforcement practices on the poor and marginalised'.

In an article in the national newspaper *The Hindustan Times*, I reflected on the general feeling of disappointment of the civil society with the outcome document and the stand taken by many developing countries including India on the role of communities and harm reduction as a strategy.

'The outcome document was the attempt to reach a consensus among highly polarised groups of countries. It fell short on several counts, most prominently on harm reduction and death penalty…… India's position on the world drug regime and the international conventions was more aligned with countries that are more in favour of the status quo and more stringent implementation of drug laws. It was a missed opportunity for the country to project its advanced policies on harm reduction'. (*Interview in Hindustan Times. 'The dose was all wrong at UN'. 2 May 2016.*)

HIGH-LEVEL MEETING ON ENDING AIDS–JUNE 2016 (UNGA POLITICAL DECLARATION TO FAST-TRACK AIDS RESPONSE)

After the highly visible SDG event in September 2015, the HLM on AIDS in June 2016 generated a lot of hope and excitement among the communities. The ambitious target of ending AIDS by 2030 needed to be disaggregated into quantifiable sub-targets with clear deadlines. Preparatory process started with UNAIDS taking the lead in organising the meeting in June 2016.

The SG's report of April 2016 issued before the HLM was a forceful appeal to member states to fast-track the response by adopting bold and ambitious targets and commit sufficient funds to achieve them. It called for front loading investments of $26 billion by 2020, ensuring 28 million adults and 1.2 million children to be put on ART, eliminate mother-to-child transmission by 2020, reduce new infections among young women to less than 100,000 by 2020, leave no one behind and ensure access to services by removing punitive laws, policies and practices that violate human rights.

The report also recommended regional fast-track targets in quantifiable terms challenging the countries to rise to the occasion and adopt them.

But the draft outcome document which would form the basis for negotiations fell short of requirements on number of key issues. As SESG I conveyed my concerns to UNAIDS on some notable omissions.

1.   There was no mention about the slowing down of the response in the past 5 years. This was emphasised in SG's report. The draft Political Declaration (PD) except for expressing concern did not mention any of these important observations.

2.   The decision of the Global Fund and other international partners to shift away from middle-income countries was highlighted in the SG's report but was completely missing in the zero draft. It was necessary that countries highlight this huge gap in funding which may become a reality from 2017. The total resource need which was quantified in the SG's report as domestic, public and international was also missing in the draft resolution.

3.   The recommendations for action contained in the SG's report were truly exceptional and some of them did find mention in the resolution. But the recommendation to ensure that at least one quarter of AIDS resources are allocated to prevention among the vulnerable populations went missing in the PD. To me that was the most important outcome we could expect from the PD to alter the course of the epidemic and response. We must ensure that it was taken on board during negotiations.

4.   There was no mention of how many countries achieved MDG 6, even though it was recognised that outstanding progress has been made on this front. There have been glaring failures also. Concern should be expressed on why so many countries failed to achieve MDG.

5.   The section on technology development was inadequately worded. There was not enough thrust on vaccine development. It was mentioned in passing, bunched with several others. We should urgently seek accelerated efforts towards development of HIV vaccines.

6.   There was a lot of emphasis on Universal Health Coverage and integration of AIDS programmes with general health, right in the

beginning. Paragraph 3 of the resolution begins with moving away from single disease to a systems approach. Are we comfortable with this? As it is an HLM on AIDS, we need to keep the focus on AIDS and talk of integration in a phased manner.

The tortuous process of negotiations got into problems while addressing the issues related to key populations, sexual and reproductive health and rights and comprehensive sexual education (CSE). These issues eluded a consensus. Some countries that were struggling with generalised epidemics felt that the term 'key populations' was not representative of the people who carry the burden of the epidemic in their setting, where young women and girls were the most vulnerable to HIV infection. CSE–as understood as an age-appropriate, culturally relevant approach to teaching about sex and relationships also ran into controversy; while some argued the necessity of such an approach to counter the HIV epidemic, others see this language as infringing their sovereignty regarding the national education curriculum. Interventions by Russia, Iran, Indonesia and a group of Gulf States have resulted in the removal of references to the need to repeal discriminatory and punitive laws affecting sex workers, people who use drugs and MSM. References to ensuring access to tailored HIV-combination prevention services for key populations were also removed and an explicit list of key populations went missing from the draft declaration.

I attended the meeting on June 8, along with my fellow envoys from CCEA and Caribbean regions with lot of expectations.

But the HLM virtually ended in a few hours after start on the first day! The PD, the core agenda of the meeting under negotiation for the past 2 months, was unanimously adopted on the first day without any discussion, leaving the large number of civil society participants and community groups in disbelief. Activists walked out in protest after the resolution was adopted on the first day of the 3-day summit, which had already been the subject of intense criticism for excluding gay and transgender organisations. More than 50 countries, including Russia, Saudi Arabia and Iran blocked community groups of sex workers, transgenders, drug users and MSM from attending the conference.

The 25-page declaration, which ran into 79 paragraphs, contained commitments addressing all sections of society vulnerable to HIV/AIDS, women, young people and adolescent girls, migrant populations and poor and marginalised communities. But nowhere in the last 27 paragraphs, which contain various global targets and commitments, was there any mention of the key affected populations–sex workers and their clients, people who use drugs and the LGBT community. (They were referred to by the generic term 'people living with, at risk of, and affected by HIV' in more than one paragraph of the declaration.)

On the positive side, the declaration successfully set quantitative targets the world community pledged to fulfil by 2020 and later by 2030. These related to (1) committing financial resources for treatment programmes to fulfil the 90-90-90 targets, (2) overseas development assistance to reach the agreed 0.7% of GDP for developed countries and (3) spending a quarter of the AIDS budgets on prevention. The commitment to put 30 million people on treatment was a commendable objective, which was expected to save the lives of 11 million people in the next 15 years and stop a further 16.5 million people from getting infected by HIV. There was strong commitment to working towards reducing sexual transmission of HIV by 50% by 2020, reducing transmission of HIV among people who inject drugs by 50% by 2020, elimination of mother-to-child transmission of HIV by 2020 and substantially reducing AIDS-related maternal deaths.

After returning to India immediately after the HLM, I shared my concerns in an opinion piece in *The Hindustan Times*.

'The much awaited High Level Meeting (HLM) on AIDS convened in United Nations, New York started on 8 June and virtually ended within a few hours after that! .... This is the second time after the UN Special Session (UNGASS) on drug use that such a resolution of far reaching implications was adopted without a debate.....

Overwhelming evidence exists on how countries have not adequately invested in prevention of new infections among these groups (LGBT Community) and how a large proportion among them are still denied access to anti-retroviral treatment (ART) because of deep rooted stigma and oppressive legal systems. But they remain unmarked and unnamed, subsumed under the name of affected populations in the Declaration.......

With no important world event planned for the next five years concerning HIV/AIDS and with ambitious targets set at the meeting, it is hard and determined work that lies ahead for countries to fulfil the commitments they have made at the meeting. Five years is not a long period in the global fight against AIDS but the next five will determine whether "Ending AIDS by 2030" is an achievable goal or will remain a distant dream.'[8]

The civil society was heartbroken. They felt thoroughly marginalised in the meeting as well as in the declaration. Some felt that the special relationship with UNAIDS of trust and collaboration was chipped irreparably.

Mona Mishra, a long-time civil society activist from India, expressed it strongly in her *Huffington Post* article.

'Two contradictory statements emerged after the adoption of the 2016 Political Declaration on HIV and AIDS by Member States of the UN at the recently concluded UNGASS last week. Michel Sidibe, EXD of UNAIDS, was quoted in the *New York Times* saying that he felt "the declaration was something to be proud of". In sharp contrast, campaigners from across the world have called the Political Declaration a "high-level failure". In a scathing statement issued by the global coalitions of civil society organizations, reflecting their disbelief and anger at the fatal omissions, they further called it "a significant set-back" and a "very weak" declaration'........

Has UNAIDS been caught napping? It is hard to believe that UNAIDS wasn't in the full know of this disaster before it unfolded.

Egypt, Iran, Saudi Arabia, Sudan, Indonesia and the Holy See, among others, made sure that the final draft of the declaration was left with the very minimum explicit mention of gay and MSM, people who use drugs, sex workers and transgender people. The heart of the HIV response was reduced to just one paragraph in a 26-page document. Member states who were disappointed with this were unable or unwilling to weigh in strongly enough to make the emphasis swing the other way.

Michel Sidibe, EXD of UNAIDS, explains this as cultural sensitivities saying, 'I think anything linked to sexuality is very complex. Is it about taboo? Is it about norms? Is it about the position of people in the society? It's about so many factors, cultural factors, economic factors. That's why AIDS is so complex. It's not easy to deal with a political declaration when you're talking about HIV/AIDS. You're confronting different societies, different opinions.

Even if mild, this is officialese for an admission of defeat.'[9]

There was a general feeling that the slowing down of global AIDS response was more to do with the new and self-defeating approach towards marginalised communities who were bearing the brunt of the epidemic. Providing treatment to infected persons was regarded as a humanitarian act and received support from all shades of political opinion. But providing affirmative support to these communities to protect themselves from getting infected and improving their social and legal status was not a matter of political consensus. Fact was that more and more countries were veering to a highly conservative view in the matter of protection of the rights including right to health of sex workers, people who use drugs, MSM and transgender populations. These were the new realities of global AIDS response post 2016. And the optimism generated after the high-profile SDG event in 2015 was short-lived specifically in the case of global response to AIDS.

INTERNATIONAL AIDS CONFERENCE, DURBAN, JULY 2016

The International AIDS Conference in Durban was the next high-profile event after the UNGASS of drugs in April and the HLM on AIDS in June 2016. Both these conferences left me disappointed that the high-level advocacy being carried out by UNAIDS and other leading advocates with countries for taking effective prevention mesaures to stop the spread of the virus was not having the desired impact on their policies governing key populations. More and more governments were opposing even to the mention of key populations in the declarations. This was a far cry from the UNGASS 2001 when the communities of key populations could effectively engage with national governments for getting a declaration which explicitily recognised their central role in the AIDS response. And its precurser, the Durban IAC of 2000 was responsible for galvanising global opinion to commit resources and prioritise AIDS responses. From 2000 to 2016 we have turned the full circle and it was like going back to the basics once again!

I was not in a mood to attend the IAC Durban which was taking place in a totally different political environment with global AIDS response showing signs of fatigue both with donor and recepient governments. Except the impressive scale-up of treatment programmes which covered 15 million persons by 2016 and the possibiity of elimination of MTCT there was nothing to write home about. The tap of new infections was leaking profusely with 1.5 million annual infections reported in 2016.

But two events motivated me to make a trip to Durban. A breakfast meeting was planned by UNDP with community representatives to interact with SG Ban Ki-moon and the SEs were asked to join the meeting. Since this will be his last AIDS conference as SG, the informal breakfast dialogue would be an opportunity for civil society to express its thanks to Ban Ki-moon for his leadership on the issues. It will also be an opportunity to discuss future priorities for civil society engagement in the AIDS response and global health more broadly. For the three of us as his SEs, that would be the last opportunity to interact with the SG and I did not want to miss it. Second was an interactive dialogue UNAIDS organised for the SEs with the communities in the Community Village in the Conference. The UNDP and International HIV/AIDS Alliance were also organising panel discussions and wanted me to join as a panelist.

The SG's breakfast meeting was an open forum where he made it very clear that without the involvement of key populationss the goal of ending AIDS will not be reached. The disappointment of civil society with the outcome of HLM in New York was discernible and they needed this conference to find their voice. We as SEs lent our support to the key populations and felt that prevention of new infections was the key to the global response and the challenge was to find sustained finances for prevention programmes among competing priorities. Eric Goosby, the SE on TB, also joined us in the interactive session with the communities which took place in the Global Village.

But I missed the activism, the fervour and the commitment which marked Durban 2000 in this IAC and returned to India.

CHANGE OF GUARD AT UNITED NATIONS

By the end of September 2016, it was clear that the former President of Portugal Antonio Guterres, would be the new SG set to assume office from 1 January 2017. All the three envoys wanted to have a structured meeting with SG Ban Ki-moon before he laid office. With the efforts of the New York Office (NYO) of UNAIDS a meeting was successfully arranged for 30 November 2016 followed by a World AIDS Day function in New York. I was happy at the opportunity to meet Ban Ki-moon to thank and bid farewell. He was a constant source of encouragement for my work as SE and greatly valued my inputs from Asia Pacific region with which he had a strong bond. We put together a summary of our work in the three regions and UNAIDS brought out a nice booklet for presentation to the SG. We met him on 30 November and presented our report. Michel and Simon Bland from NYO were also present. In my summary note I expressed concern at the waning of global interest in AIDS programmes and marginalisation of key populations.

'During this period, in international and regional meetings such as the 21st International AIDS Conference in Durban in June 2016, the 2016 High-Level Meeting on Ending AIDS and the United Nations General Assembly Special Session (UNGASS) on Drugs, I took the opportunity to reach out to community leaders of key populations and people living with HIV. I have sensed a growing resentment and despondency among many who feel that their relevance in global response to AIDS is diminishing. The absence of explicit mention in the Political Declaration at the High-Level Meeting and the failure to mention harm reduction in the UNGASS resolution on drugs have been demoralizing for communities who were expecting that their central role in the AIDS response would be acknowledged by national governments. Increasing stringency of national laws governing drug use and same-sex relations in many countries is a disturbing trend and a cause of worry for civil society. The Philippines presents the worst case, where the newly elected leadership has declared an open war on drugs.

Participation in civil society programmes and expressing solidarity with their cause will continue to be areas of priority for the UNSE. It will be necessary to keep sharp focus in coming years on policies and programmes in the region, with high impact in both reducing new infections and in saving the lives of people who are living with HIV. Middle-income countries, which account for bulk of new infections, will face funding shortage from external sources. They need to find domestic resources to fill the resource gap which needs evidence-based advocacy'. (*Report of the UN Special Envoys to Secretary-General Ban Ki-moon, 30 November 2016*)

SG Ban Ki-moon was pleasant and informal in his conversation and appreciated our work in the regions. It was a touching moment for us ending 5 years of an association which was exciting and fulfilling. For me, it was a great moment for ending my 20 years of association with AIDS programmes, first in the Government of India and later in the UN system—in UNAIDS and with the SG for past 5 years.

After my return to India, Steve Kraus, the RD, welcomed me to Bangkok on 6 December to a debriefing with the UN regional focal points on AIDS, development partners and regional CSO representatives. I touched upon my work in the region in the past 5 years, identified the challenges and made a few suggestions on way forward. I thanked Steve and my point persons in the RST, Marlyn Borromeo and Gaye Watchareeporn for the tremendous support they provided all these years. They all gave me an affectionate farewell at the end.

As I returned to Bangalore I got an urgent message from Geneva that the new SG designate wanted to know if I would be willing to continue as SE for some time. I was surprised as I thought the new SG would choose his own team to support him. I assumed that he must be looking at it as a transition arrangement and conveyed my assent. I presented a tentative plan of work which included possible missions to Philippines and Indonesia and a meeting with Health Minister, India.

Something unforeseen happened in February 2017. I had to undergo a spinal surgery when the acute lower back pain I was managing for a few years became unbearable. I was in the hospital for a couple of days only but was advised not to travel for the next 2 months. I cancelled all my travel plans to Bangkok, Manila and Delhi and stayed back in Bangalore, recovering from the postoperative effects of the surgery.

May 2017 was an important milestone in my career as a civil servant. I along with my IAS and civil services colleagues who joined the service in 1967 were completing 50 years and a golden jubilee meet was organised by the Lal Bahadur Shastri National Academy of Administration at Mussoorie, a hill station in the foothills of Himalayas where we as young trainees underwent our induction training for 1 year. My wife and I did not want to miss the event and travelled to Mussoorie to spend 3 engaging days in the company of my former service colleagues and their spouses, some of whom we met for the first time after 50 years! We lived through the memorable moments of the past five decades and that was the best way for me to bounce back into activity. Coming 3 months after my surgery it was also a test check for my health in the postrecovery phase.

But the 3 months of interregnum did not work out well for arranging country missions to Philippines and Indonesia as originally planned. Number of administrative changes took place in UNAIDS. Indonesia had a new UCD, Tina Boonto who worked earlier as a programme advisor in Myanmar. She was settling down and it was too premature to undertake a mission. At the regional level, Steve Kraus was retiring in June 2017 and Eamonn Murphy was appointed as the new RST Director. In the middle of so many transitions occurring during the period, I thought it was not advisable for me to plan a country visit.

In June, UNAIDS Geneva decided to invite the three envoys to the 40th meeting of PCB on 28 and 29 June 2017, as Observers. By then it was clear that the new SG would not be having envoys for HIV/AIDS and we would be laying down office by end of June. It was the last occasion for us to share our thoughts with the policy-making body of UNAIDS and bid farewell to the EXD and the senior management of the joint UN programme. I attended the PCB on 28th and 29th and shared my concerns on the state of regional response to AIDS in Asia Pacific. What I said in the meeting holds good even today and worth reproducing here.

'Working closely with country leadership in Asia Pacific region, I feel concerned at the decline of AIDS as a political priority. Early successes in containing the epidemic and the steady reduction in mortality have created an impression that the battle against AIDS has already been won and only the last rites remain to be performed. Global advocacy for taking AIDS out of isolation and mainstreaming it into health systems should not lead us to the conclusion that the need for focused AIDS interventions is over. We are seeing global public opinion alternating between the two extremes of AIDS exceptionalism and complete mainstreaming, both of which are not realistic approaches to AIDS control.

We still have enormous challenges at country level: rising infection rates in a number of countries coupled with increasingly adverse legal environment are making the task of controlling the epidemic more and more difficult. We need to have a conversation with country leadership on how essential a friendly legal environment is for a successful national response. When a HIV+ UN staff member working in Uganda has been driven to such desperation that she decided to end her life without accessing treatment, it clearly shows that the battle to end stigma is not being won.

We should not also depart from established evidence that the key populations are central to AIDS response in Asia Pacific. The slow decrease in incidence to almost zero levels should make us all worried. This trend can't be reversed unless we achieve significant coverage levels of the key populations with prevention and treatment interventions. It is also wrong to think that the same targeted approach will work for all the important key population groups. We need to make our programmes tailor made to the needs of various population groups based on their behaviours and vulnerabilities.

It is heartening to see countries in Asia invest more and more of their domestic resources into AIDS programmes. But a significant part of these resources need to flow into high impact prevention among the key populations to make a meaningful impact in bringing down the incidence rates in the next few years.

The report of the Global Review Panel should also enable the participating agencies in the joint UN programme to take a hard look at their own effectiveness in performing the roles assigned to them under the division of labour a decade ago.

As I take leave as the SE of UNSG on AIDS, I like to thank the former SG Mr. Ban Ki-moon, the present SG Mr. Antonio Guterres and Michel for the confidence they reposed in me to be the advocate for ending AIDS in Asia Pacific. Before concluding, I want to leave this simple thought with you. **Please tell the world that AIDS is not over! Not yet. And countries which have set for themselves the task of ending AIDS by 2030 should not rest until it is over.'**

I was also invited to attend the thematic segment of the PCB the next day. In my intervention I tried to identify issues hindering effective prevention at country and regional levels. The most important issue was the shrinking legal space for civil society and rising fundamentalism impacting upon key populations which need to be addressed in the 33 fast-track countries. The joint UN programme need to speak forcefully with country leadership to make, at least the law on the streets more friendly to the key populations to facilitate their access to prevention programmes. Law enforcement should get greater emphasis for immediate benefits.

I highlighted the following issues as critical which should find priority in the work of the prevention group in the secretariat.

1. Prevention benefits are not immediate, tangible and not directly measurable unlike the treatment and PMTCT programmes. We need to employ indirect methods to measure the impact of prevention programmes such as the infections averted over a period of time. Many countries do not do it due to lack of capacity. We need to ask our Strategic Information Division to devise methodologies of estimating averted infections due to prevention interventions and create capacity at country level to undertake these measurements at least once in 3 years. This data can be a powerful advocacy tool for scaling up prevention programmes in fast-track countries.

2. We are aware that prevention is not a biomedical intervention. The powerful medical lobby, the health systems and the pharmaceutical industry do not feel involved in prevention work. It is time we get them on board and make them speak for prevention. In many countries they

have powerful influence on governments and can be effective advocates for prevention of new infections as it makes good public health sense.

3. Our communication strategy around prevention should bring back the importance of primary prevention tools such as condoms and safe needles. The new technologies for example pre-exposure prophylaxis (PreP), male circumcision and female microbicides are not standalone prevention tools and need to be used in conjunction with the traditional tools such as condoms and safe needles.

I thought I must share my concern about the division of labour within the UN cosponsors on the prevention agenda and spoke out my mind. I said, 'within the cosponsors, prevention is dispersed among four or five agencies based on key populations without any horizontal coordination. The key populations are not watertight groups and overlap a lot. A sex worker can also inject drugs and a drug user can also be an MSM or transgender. We are not effectively addressing this overlap within the cosponsors. As secretariat, you have a coordination function to bring these agencies together and report on what they are doing on prevention instead of on individual groups'.

The last point was one that always troubled me ever since the division of labour between cosponsors and secretariat was announced in 2006. Effective remedies could not be found by the joint programme ever since for rectifying this weakness.

Next day, Michel arranged an affectionate farewell for the three envoys, Steve Kraus and Sheila Talou, the Regional Directors of Asia Pacific and Eastern and Southern Africa who were also demitting office. I left Geneva and my assignment as SE to UNSG with a good feeling of fulfilment. Coming at the end of my tenure as RD UNAIDS, the SE assignment was a rare opportunity of working on high-level advocacy with countries and interacting with the SG and senior UN officials in the joint UN programme.

But the last word was still not said on my involvement with AIDS responses. In the PCB meeting Michel announced that he would like me and Eddie Greene, SE for Caribbean, to work with UNAIDS for another 6 months in an advisory capacity to support the regions (Asia Pacific and Caribbean) and the prevention group in Geneva for advocating on the importance of prevention in challenging countries. However, it took Geneva 3 months to work out the modalities of such involvement in an advisory role. Finally we agreed that I would undertake two high-level review missions to India and Indonesia during last quarter of 2017 and finish my assignment.

INDIA MISSION

Eamonn was keen to do a joint mission with me of both these countries. After ascertaining the convenience of the host governments, we did a 3-day mission to India from 30 October to 2 November, 2017. After meeting senior officials of health ministry and NACO in Delhi we paid a 1-day visit to Mumbai to interact with the Municipal Commissioner of Mumbai and the PDs of Mumbai and Maharashtra SACS. I did not get an occasion to take a close look at India's AIDS response for a couple of years now and what I saw on the ground was a worrisome situation of slowing down of prevention activities among the key populations. The Municipal Commissioner of Mumbai, a senior civil servant from IAS, was enquiring whether AIDS was still a living issue in India necessitating a UN high level mission! I had to appraise him of the declining focus on AIDS response and the threat of resurgence in numbers if timely action was not taken. He pointed out to the lack of visibility of the programme giving an impression that it was no more a serious public health issue. I was surprised at this reaction from a very senior government functionary and got convinced that over the past few years HIV/AIDS slipped out of public memory and an entire generation of young people grew up without even basic knowledge of the risks of HIV/AIDS. The NACP IV suffered from inadequate allocation of resources right from the beginning and even the sanctioned allocations were not always available for the programme. It was extended until March 2020 which prevented a new phase of response, the NACP V coming into operation. The meeting with civil society partners exposed the deep chasm between the government and civil society.

My impression after the mission was that India's AIDS response was at a critical juncture. In the past it was one of the most comprehensive national programmes in the world, implemented by a committed set of professionals at the central and state level with participation of civil society and vulnerable communities. The results were there to see. But the slowing down of the response in the past few years was a matter of great concern. At its current level, there was little likelihood of the stiff fast-track targets for 2020 being achieved. We pointed to the urgent need for the government to act, by approving the new National Strategic Plan 2017-2022, by committing full funding to all components of the programme, addressing governance and convergence issues and once again opening doors to civil society to participate meaningfully. It was time to brush up public memory about AIDS and its disastrous consequences by launching an ambitious IEC campaign in the country bringing out the risks of complacency.

I have devoted space in the last chapter for a more detailed evaluation of India's AIDS response and what was ailing it.

INDONESIA MISSION

The Indonesia mission, the last job on my hands, was plagued by many problems of nonavailability of dates and had to be postponed to 2018. After serious efforts I could do that along with Eamonn Murphy in March 2018. Tina Bantoo was well settled as UCD and prepared a detailed programme for us.

In Asia and the Pacific Region, Indonesia contributes significantly to the overall HIV burden. It has the third highest number of new HIV infections after India and China at an annual estimate of 48,000 people. Without rapid scale-up of effective prevention programmes, the number of people living with HIV can in a few years surpass 1 million (from the current estimate of 630,000 people living with HIV as at 2017). During the mission, we discussed the issues and challenges of the HIV response in Indonesia with senior-level functionaries both in government and nongovernment sectors. We met with the Deputy Coordinating Minister for Human Development & Culture; Ministry of Health's Director General of Disease Control; the Vice Governor of DKI Jakarta; the Chair of the Global Fund Country Coordinating Mechanism (CCM) and international development partners.

One big setback we noticed since our last visit in 2015 was the phasing out of the National AIDS Commission which was active under the leadership of Ibu Nafsiah in the earlier years. The Coordinating Ministry for Human Development & Culture was given the responsibility of providing leadership on strategic guidance and coordinating with the provincial governments.

Low coverage of interventions for prevention and treatment explains the fast rise of new infections. Only 30% of estimated people living with HIV (PLHIV) knew their status. This was a critical barrier to scaling-up HIV prevention, care and treatment interventions. Only 13% of the estimated 630,000 PLHIV could access ARV treatment as against the target of 75% coverage by 2020 which was just 2 years down the line. National programmes on prevention of HIV through sexual transmission were getting undermined by the closure of brothels across the country. We were also concerned that the harm reduction programmes were getting impacted by a punitive approach to drug use. Of particular concern, was the new criminal code amendment that may undermine the HIV response by adopting a punitive approach to community-based services on HIV.

On the positive side, the inclusion of HIV in the Minimum Standard of Services (SPM-MMS) policy by the Ministry of Home Affairs was a good development which will set working indicators to measure performance of sub-national governments in providing basic services to its citizens. Indonesia could keep the HIV prevalence at a low level. But prevalence does not tell the whole story. It was the incidence, that is, number of new infections which need to be reduced to 10% of the present level if the globally agreed targets are to be met. But currently they are on the rise. We left a set of recommendations with the government in an aide memoir.

I was particularly worried about the disbanding of NAC which went against the three ones principle–the basic framework for national responses. During the last mission we did in Indonesia in October 2015 we in fact recommended strengthening the NAC governance and providing them with more funds. Altogether disbanding it was sure to hurt the national AIDS response in Indonesia which together with Pakistan and Philippines would be the most challenging countries for realisation of the stiff fast-track targets for 2020.

I stopped for a day in Bangkok during my return to meet the RST team to bid them goodbye one last time and thank them for the wonderful support they provided during all those years of my work in the UN system.

REFERENCES

1. UN solution to AIDS muddled. *Bangkok Post* 31 July; 2012. Available at: https://www.bangkokpost.com/opinion/opinion/305113/un-solution-to-aids-muddled

2. United Nations; Office on Drugs and Crime. 2012 International AIDS Conference. Washington DC. Available at: https://www.unodc.org/unodc/en/frontpage/2012/July/2012-international-aids-conference-opens-in-washington-dc.html

3. Rao JVRP, Separating consent from exploitation. *Hindustan Times* 2013. Available at: https://www.hindustantimes.com/india/separating-consent-from-exploitation/story-2qFA7x88VeRduRWkYyAKXI.html

4. Nishtar S, Mehboob AB. Pakistan prepares to abolish Ministry of Health. *Lancet* 2011;378(9792):648-649.

5. Gaviria C. President Duterte is repeating my mistakes. Op-Ed. *The New York Times* February 7, 2017.

6. United Nations. General Assembly. Report of the Secretary-General: Implementation of the Declaration of Commitment on HIV/AIDS and the Political Declaration on HIV/AIDSUniting for universal access: towards zero new HIV infections, zero discrimination and zero AIDS-related deaths. Sixty-Fifth Session. 2011. Available at: https://files.unaids.org/en/media/unaids/contentassets/documents/document/2011/A-65-797_English.pdf

7. United Nations. General Assembly. Report of the Secretary General: Resolution adopted by the General Assembly on 10 April 2014. Improving Global Road Safety. Sixty-Eighth Session 68/269. 2014. Available at: https://www.un.org/en/ga/search/view_doc.asp?symbol=A/RES/68/269&referer=http://www.un.org/en/ga/68/resolutions.shtml&Lang=E

8. RAO JVRP. The UNAIDS declaration on eradication is a half-done job. Article in *Hindustan Times*. June 23, 2016. Available at: https://www.hindustantimes.com/analysis/the-unaids-declaration-on-eradication-is-a-half-done-job/story-aa5FPDCIM8LkoG7EsPZbbP.html

9. Mishra M. Why UNAIDS's 'Bold New Declaration' is a travesty. *HUFFPOST* 2016. Available at: *http://www.huffingtonpost.in/mona-mishra/why-unaidss-bold-new-decl_b_10584370.html*

CHAPTER 5

WORKING WITH CIVIL SOCIETY

By not opting for a regular 9 to 5 job after leaving Bangkok in 2010, I could involve myself more in civil society work with organisations working on broader public health issues apart from HIV/AIDS. I had to manage my time judiciously for keeping a proper work–life balance and factor in the long travel time to Delhi while working with Delhi-based organisations and the Government of India. I had joined the Boards of two nongovernmental organisations (NGOs) based in Bangalore–Swasti and Centre for Budget Policy and Control (CBPC) as honorary member and provided strategic support on policy and programming. On the global front I got involved with two organisations well known for their contribution to global public health–the International HIV/AIDS Alliance (IHAA) in Brighton, United Kingdom, and the Institute of Health Matrices and Evaluation (IHME) in Seattle, United States.

INTERNATIONAL HIV/AIDS ALLIANCE AND THE INDIA LINKING ORGANISATION

After my return to India in 2010, Bai Bagasao my long-time colleague and the UNAIDS Country Coordinator in the Philippines, informed me she was on the Board of Trustees of IHAA in Brighton and would be rotating out after completing her tenure. The IHAA was looking for a new director on their board from Asia. Bai encouraged me to offer my candidature as the appointment of trustees was through an application process. I sent my curriculum vitae and was shortlisted. Nafis Sadik, the Special Envoy of Secretary-General (SESG) was also on the Board and encouraged me to join. I was invited to join the International Board in November 2010 and continued until 2019.

Established in 1993, the IHAA is a global partnership of nationally based organisations working to support community action on AIDS in developing countries. A network of independent, locally governed linking organisations (LOs) work as intermediaries; while they might provide some direct services, their main objective was to assist other groups responding to HIV. In some countries IHAA has established country offices which are governed by IHAA's international secretariat but led and staffed by nationals. An accreditation system had been designed to guarantee high institutional and programmatic standards, as assessed by peer review for the LOs.

Recently the organisation changed its name to 'Frontline AIDS' to more strongly reflect its commitment to lead the fight against AIDS and for the rights of infected and affected communities. The Frontline AIDS secretariat is governed by a Board of Trustees which approves the global strategy and is responsible for ensuring that the organisation's broad policies and strategies are in keeping with its mission.

Frontline AIDS has a strong presence in all regions and connected with the field through the LOs. It also has branch offices in countries such as India and Cambodia, which were progressively converted into LOs with independent boards. India office was going through this transition when I joined the Alliance. I was asked to join the India Board as a member and later as the Chair when it became a fully Indian LO. Apart from contributing to the Board decisions in IHAA, I was given the responsibility of handholding the India Board by inducting new members and recruiting an Indian Executive Director in keeping with the policy of autonomous governance of the LOs.

In 2015, the IHAA Board took a decision that a board member should not hold a parallel position in a national LO to avoid possible conflict of interest. I left the India Board in 2016 after recruiting the new Executive Director, Sonal Mehta, and passing on the Board leadership to S.Y. Quraishi who joined the board earlier as a member.

The India HIV/Alliance is a strong NGO with close links with India's national programme and could access sustained financial support from Global Fund for programmes such as *Pehchan* and *Vihaan* providing community support to government-led interventions for treatment and prevention.

I enjoyed my work in IHAA which was professionally well run with good financial systems and controls. The Board chairs, Steven Sinding and Martin Dinham, were men of high professional competence and integrity and held the Board and the secretariat together with their leadership qualities. Alvaro Bermijo, the Executive Director, and his successor Christine Stegling provided great leadership to the organisation in Brighton, United Kingdom, and across the LOs and country offices.

Like many INGOs, IHAA also faced financial challenges with many of the traditional donors either reducing or withdrawing organisational support given as unlinked funding. The global gag rule on anti-abortion introduced by United States resulted in deprivation of funding from that country. The global gag rule prohibits foreign NGOs who receive US global health assistance from providing legal abortion services or referrals, while also barring advocacy for abortion law reform–even if it's done with the NGO's own, non-US funds. In 2017, President Donald Trump's Protecting Life in Global Health Assistance policy expanded the global gag rule, applying it to recipients of any US global health funding, totaling an unprecedented $8.8 billion. Everything from HIV/AIDS programming and health systems strengthening to programmes that support water, sanitation, and hygiene were negatively impacted. The policy allows access to abortion only in cases of rape, incest or when a woman's life is at risk. The IHAA Board deliberated on the option and stood its ground by not agreeing to sign the declaration. Other European donors such as Swedish International Development Cooperation Agency (SIDA) came forward to fill the gap. The organisation had to go through a process of rationalisation of staff structure to meet fund shortage. But the strength of the Alliance were its LOs who implement programmes and provide field-level feedback to the organisation for constant evaluation of its strategy.

INSTITUTE OF HEALTH MATRICES AND EVALUATION (IHME) AND DISEASE BURDEN STUDIES

In 2011, Peter Piot wrote to me that he would be chairing an Independent Advisory Committee (IAC) for the IHME located in Seattle, United States, and asked me to join the group. The Independent Advisory Committee for the Global Burden of Disease (GBD) studies would advise the Board of the IHME and the Director on GBD, forecasting and geospatial analysis research areas. While the committee would mostly be having experts in epidemiology and disease surveillance, Peter wanted to include members from developing countries who have experience in implementing public health programmes at national level. I and Fatima Marinho, from Brazil, represented this group of country programmers and Irene Agyepong from Kenya joined us later. The 12-member Committee met for the first time in November 2013 in Brussels in the offices of King Bedouin Foundation who were providing logistic support to the Committee's work and got a detailed briefing on IHME, its mandate and its work on GBD studies. Members suggested among other things, improvement of the project's communications strategy to address some of the criticisms over transparency; ensuring that the new plans for GBD work remain within the scope of the project and the IHME team. For me it was a totally new group and except for Peter I was meeting most of the other members for the first time.

From the second meeting, the Committee started holding its biannual meetings in IHME at Seattle, which provided us an opportunity to meet its research groups and understand its way of working. As we progressed, I realised the immense potential the GBD estimations possess in influencing decision making at country level on investments in health sector programmes. The Institute was publishing sub-national estimates for United Kingdom, China and Mexico and wanted to bring in more countries such as India and Brazil into this programme. The scientific excellence and technical soundness of the study results made its annual publication in the *Lancet* a much sought after storehouse of information among researchers in public health. I was more excited about the use of the disease burden study and estimations at sub-national level to inform and influence policies and investments at provincial level in the developing countries. I got closely involved with the work of sub-national estimates for India which was getting organised in collaboration with Public Health Foundation of India (PHFI) and Indian Council of Medical Research (ICMR). Lalit Dandona, from PHFI, was the point person for sub-national estimate preparation in India. I chaired a national-level advisory body constituted to coordinate the effort. There were initial hiccups because of the reluctance of Registrar General of India to share mortality data with the GBD programme. The agency got on board after the significance of the study and its potential to influence policy were explained to them. We started preparing for a national release of the estimates for India simultaneously with their publication in *Lancet* in November 2017.

The IAC met in Delhi during the launch of the sub-national estimates for India and many of the IAC members attended the national event. There was high-profile participation of Indian Government and the states in the function. The Health Minister, Minister of State and Member, Health of NITI Aayog (which replaced the Planning Commission of India) were present at the launch. Many state representatives also participated in the event. The Vice President of India launched the report and the media extensively covered the results. The IAC commended IHME, PHFI and ICMR on their breakthrough collaborations and the successful launch of the state-level burden of disease study in India. The IAC also noted the importance of continued engagement with various Indian stakeholders to ensure the long-term success of the initiative.

I could foresee that the dissemination of findings and deliberations at this event would lead to a vibrant and even more extensive next phase of work including production of state-level disease burden estimates annually in India. This would enable understanding of the evolving trends of disease burden over time and the impact of major health interventions. Application of the state-level disease burden findings has the potential to inform policy, to monitor sustainable development goals and to forecast population health under various scenarios in each state of India.

Brazil also had an impressive record of collaboration on GBD studies and was preparing sub-national estimates. In November 2018, the IAC met in Rio where the members were invited to attend the Second Scientific

Meeting of GBD Brazil Project, organised by the Brazilian Burden of Disease (BoD) network. The network presented the history, objectives, experience and on-going BoD research across Brazil, supported by the Brazilian Ministry of Health. Members of the IAC were unanimous in their appreciation of the lessons shared by the highly organised network.

The IHME entered into a memorandum of understanding (MOU) with WHO under the new Director General and a WHO representative now sits on the IAC for ensuring close collaboration between the two agencies. The IAC regularly reviews the partnership between IHME and WHO under the MOU.

In November 2019, the IAC meeting at Singapore brought into focus the importance of 'precision public health' a new buzzword doing rounds for the past couple of years. The NUS School of Public Health, Singapore, felt that by mixing the technical advancements of precision medicine with the goals of public health, practitioners of precision public health can improve health at the population level. While many think of precision public health as the application of public health measures to individuals, at the NUS School of Public Health precision public health was perceived to work at three levels: individual, community and health system as well as global. They see a critical role for GBD in the application of precision public health worldwide. The Singapore example shows how GBD can be used to inform what governments and ministries of health in Asian countries should focus on. The IAC is expected to examine this further in future meetings of the Committee.

PUBLIC HEALTH FOUNDATION OF INDIA (PHFI)

I described my involvement in the PHFI in Chapter 1. After my retirement as Health Secretary in December 2004, the Foundation was finally established in 2006 as a registered society under the Society Registration Act 1860 with a governing council (GC) to manage its affairs. Rajat Gupta from McKinseys was elected as the Chair and Srinath Reddy was hired as the President and chief executive officer (CEO) of the organisation. I was nominated as a member representing the UN system in the Council. The Government of India was represented through the Secretary to Prime Minister, Secretary

Health, Directorate General of Health Services (DGHS) and DG ICMR. The Government of India made a major contribution of Rs. 650 million and Bill and Melinda Gates Foundation (BMGF) was the major contributor from private sector. Number of smaller private foundations also joined the initiative. The PHFI was the first major public private partnership initiative in the area of public health in India and received political support at the top level from the government. The Foundation was formally inaugurated by Prime Minister Manmohan Singh in March 2006.

For the next 4 years I could not keep close touch with the affairs of the Foundation except participating in the GC meetings whenever I had an opportunity to visit Delhi. But I always used to remind the GC about the core mandate of starting centres of excellence to impart quality public health education at postgraduate level and promote research of international standards. The Foundation started identifying possible sites for locating schools of public health and came up with five priority sites, Ahmedabad in Gujarat, Hyderabad in Andhra Pradesh (now Telangana), Delhi in northern region, Bhubaneshwar in Odisha and Shillong in North East. The state governments were willing to provide land on long-term lease for establishment of the institutes. Proposals moved fast in case of Ahmedabad, Hyderabad and Bhubaneshwar while Delhi government could not provide land which was encumbrance-free. These four institutes started functioning from rented premises with number of diploma courses in allied public health disciplines. Our plan to start Master of Public Health (MPH) degree could not progress further because of affiliation problems with the universities. Our first priority was to get PHFI recognised as a deemed university enabling award of MPH degrees to the schools affiliated to it. The proposal hit a roadblock with Human Resource Development Ministry and University Grants Commission who were reluctant to approve any more cases of deemed universities in India.

When I returned to Delhi in 2010 after my tenure in UNAIDS, I picked up the threads but found the governance structure of PHFI quite unmanageable. As a registered society it should have had a two-tier structure of a general body and a GC/board but the organisation was functioning with a large and unmanageable GC. It was not a proper forum to discuss management issues that were vital for the functioning of the organisation. At the request of the chair of the GC, I headed a governance reforms committee in 2011 and suggested a two-tier structure with a general body consisting of all members of the Foundation and a 15-member executive committee (EC) to manage its affairs. A Finance Committee, an Audit Committee and a Resource Mobilisation Committee were also proposed as a part of the reform package. The recommendations were accepted and new governance structures were established by amendment of rules in October 2011.

The IIPHs at Gandhinagar and Hyderabad were established in 2008, IIPH Delhi in 2009 and Bhubaneshwar Institute in 2010. The Gandhinagar institute later got transformed into an autonomous body with its own Board of management and its independent campus in 2017. The last one in Shillong was established in 2015. It was not until 2015 that the first MPH programmes could be started at IIPH Gandhinagar and Hyderabad. Integrated M.Sc. and Ph.D. in Health Informatics and Clinical Research were started in 2013 and a full-time Ph.D. in Health Sciences and Public Health started in IIPH Delhi in 2017. A number of postgraduate diploma courses are conducted by all institutes for both in-house health service personnel as well as freshers from the market.

When everything was going well for PHFI, it was rocked by several problems unforeseen and beyond its control which affected its functioning. Rajat Gupta, the founder chair of the Foundation, had to resign in 2011 after he was convicted in a US court on charges of insider trading. The new chair Venugopal Reddy, the former governor of Reserve Bank of India (RBI), saw the transition through and facilitated establishment of the EC, GB and other committees on the recommendation of the governance reforms committee. But he also had to leave after getting appointed as the new Chair of the Finance Commission, a constitutional body appointed once in 5 years to determine centre–state financial allocations in India.

The PHFI was fortunate to get N.R. Narayana Murthy, Founder Chairman of Infosys, the Bangalore-based IT giant as its chair in July 2011. Murthy continued to steer the organisation with his no-nonsense approach and financial prudence for the next 7 years with a brief interregnum from February 2014 to February 2015. He took a quick review of the financial situation and strongly advised that PHFI should not enter into any more agreements for IIPHs in other states because of financial constraints. After the initial spurt of resource mobilisation until 2011, very little was added to the kitty through corporate funding. The Government of India also did not provide any further grant after the initial contribution of Rs. 650 million. The sense of realism Narayana Murthy brought to the management of PHFI helped in consolidation of the mandate and work of the organisation.

But in 2014 PHFI became a victim of a banking scam involving major public sector banks in Mumbai where its funds were invested in fixed deposits. The scam involved some senior managers of the banks and funds of PHFI along with some public undertakings of Maharashtra Government were withdrawn with their connivance and involvement. Overnight the organisation was thrown into a financial turmoil as it could not access its funds invested in these banks. PHFI had to depend on its projects income to sustain itself and maintain its technical and operational strength in the headquarters and the institutes.

In April 2017, came the second blow when the license under Foreign Contributions Regulation Act (FCRA) which enabled the organisation to access external funding to undertake projects was cancelled by the government without assigning any reason. Even the funds in the pipeline for ongoing projects were frozen. These two developments coming in quick succession forced a grave existential crisis for PHFI. The leadership provided by Narayana Murthy as the Board chair, the courage and commitment of Srinath Reddy and consistent moral support by the health ministry helped the organisation to stay afloat with a shoe string budget and a highly depleted but dedicated technical and research staff.

In July 2018, Narayana Murthy left the organisation after serving his full term and handed over the reins to S. Ramadorai, a former Vice President of Tata Consultancy Services (TCS) who joined the PHFI and assumed leadership. In 2019, I finished my term as EC member and wanted to leave. But I was asked to stay as a special invitee to the EC in my capacity as the Chair of the Advisory Committee of the Delhi IIPH.

Because of consistent efforts of Srinath Reddy and the support of health ministry, some of the rigors of cancellation of FCRA were relaxed and foreign collaboration projects were getting approved on a case-to-case basis. But the organisation is still grappling with the financial crisis it was thrown into after suspension of its Foreign Contributions Regulation Act (FCRA) license. The funds involved in the banking scam were still locked up in endless court cases right up to Supreme Court and recovery proceedings. The organisation lost number of valued technical staff as external projects virtually ground to a halt during the past 2 years. The Board decided on decentralizing governance to the Institute level and grant them greater autonomy. I chaired a Board subcommittee which recommended greater autonomy to the Institutes of Public Health established in Hyderabad, Delhi, Bhubaneshwar and Shillong by registering them as autonomous societies with independent boards of management to raise resources and make the Institutes self-reliant. If this can be successfully accomplished, PHFI will be able to shed much of its financial burden and devote scarce resources to maintaining a lean and efficient head office in Delhi to perform oversight functions. The Hyderabad institute has since been registered as an autonomous society for governance but retains its close link with PHFI headquarters, much like the Gandhinagar institute.

But I have great hope that PHFI will survive all these adversities and bounce back as the premier public health institution in India. Public Health Foundation in 15 years of its existence has directly contributed to the emergence of quality public health education through its schools in Gandhinagar, Hyderabad and Delhi. Indirectly its emergence on the Indian scene also stimulated interest in public health education as an academic activity and not as an adjunct to medical schools, where it remained as a last priority for specialisation for medical graduates. When PHFI came into existence there were just two or three PH schools awarding MPH degrees in India. Today there are more than 30 of them functioning both in public and private sector. Public health education was thrown open to non-medical graduates also, thanks to the National Health Policy of 2002. What is needed now is a degree of uniformity in quality and standards across diverse schools established under different management structures. A self-regulatory mechanism on the lines of the American Association of Schools of Public Health (ASPH) would help bring in uniformity in academic and research standards across the institutes.

Finding employment for public health graduates is also critical if schools of public health have to flourish in India. Unlike management education where bulk of employment opportunities exists in private sector, it is the government which should emerge as the largest employer for public health graduates and rightly so. If government decides to spend an increasing share of its GDP as public expenditure on health, it requires a specialised cadre of public health professionals at the national and state levels to manage its programmes and institutions. PHFI played a huge advocacy role with the former Planning Commission and Ministry of Health to give priority to public health education and creation of employment opportunities to public health professionals. The National Health Policy 2017 recommended that states should establish dedicated cadres of public health professionals to manage the large number of public health programmes and health care institutions. Some states such as Tamil Nadu have since established separate public health cadres but it is still work in progress in other states. The Government of India should set an example and lead from the front by constituting a separate cadre of public health professionals to manage public health programmes initiated at national level.

JODHPUR SCHOOLS OF PUBLIC HEALTH

After my return from Bangkok, I got in touch with a team of public health professionals led by Dr. Anil Purohit, a long-time friend from my NACO days, who was engaged in establishing new schools of public health in Jodhpur and Jaipur in Rajasthan. Anil Purohit is now the Director of Global Affairs in the Bedford Stem Cells Research Foundation in Boston, United States. He founded the Jodhpur School of Public Health (JSPH) and got it affiliated to the National University of Jodhpur for the MPH degree. Over the years, JSPH has become a centre of excellence in offering training and capacity development in rural public health, drug policy and human rights, tobacco control and nutrition. Apart from Indian students the school attracted a number of foreign students who were deputed for training in public health education and research. I was invited by Anil Purohit to join as a visiting faculty and deliver talks on selective subjects of public health on suitable occasions. I could not do it regularly due to my work as the Special Envoy of UNSG but visited the JSPH when time permitted and delivered talks on subjects ranging from health policy to disease burden studies. It was a refreshing change to indulge in academic work which helped in refreshing my memory on public health policy issues and in interacting with MPH students.

In 2012 at the 20th International AIDS Conference in Washington DC, JSPH presented me with the Lifetime Contribution Award in the Field of HIV/AIDS.

In September 2013, I got a message from Anil that the university had decided to honour me with D.Litt for distinguished service in public health along with a few others from various fields of knowledge. When I heard that it would be Dr. Rangarajan and Dr. Srinath Reddy who were the other awardees, I readily agreed. On reaching Jodhpur for the function which involved an 8-hour bus journey from Jaipur because of flight cancellations, I heard that Amitabh Bachchan, the famous Bollywood legend and film personality would also be one of the awardees. The Big B, as he was called, is an institution in himself and stole the limelight at the convocation where the awards were presented. It was a great recognition for me to get an award from an academic institution for the services I rendered mostly for the government and UN system.

Anil Purohit later established the branch of JSPH at Poornima University in Jaipur, and continued to invite me to their academic programmes for MPH students. I was invited to the inauguration of the School in July 2019. I was appointed as National Professor at JSPH and the Board of Advisors at JSPH in Jaipur and Jodhpur.

VOLUNTARY HEALTH ASSOCIATION OF INDIA

VHAI is a federation of 27 state voluntary health associations and is one of the largest health and development networks in India. The association sponsors innovative health and development programmes at the grassroots level with active participation of the people. Since its establishment in 1970, VHAI strived to build up a strong health movement in the country for a cost-effective, preventive, promotive and rehabilitative health care system.

After my return to India, Dr. Alok Mukhopadhyay, the Chair of VHAI, invited me to join the Independent Commission on Development and Health (ICDHI) set up by the association in 1995 with distinguished persons from the health and development sectors in India. The Commission aims at periodically assessing the development and health situation of the country through policy research and analysis with development workers, policy makers and community leaders. The Commission members included some of my former colleagues in Health Ministry, Javid Chowdhury, Shailaja Chandra, S.Y. Quraishi, Deepak Gupta and Dr. L.M. Nath, former Director of All India Institute of Medical Sciences, Delhi. Dr. Darshan Shankar, Vice Chancellor Institute of Trans-Disciplinary Health Sciences and Technology, Bangalore, and Dr. Amit Roy, Professor of Economics from Jawaharlal Nehru University are the other members. Dr. Alok Mukhopadhyay is the Convener of the Commission.

The Commission deliberations were quite stimulating, conducted in an informal and collegial atmosphere. Working together, we brought out number of publications from the ICDHI. Prominent among them are *Keeping the Promise – two decades of India's fight against AIDS* in 2011, *A road map for India's Health* in 2015 and a paper proposing a scheme for restructuring the Ministry of Health and Family Welfare based on its mandate and functions to deal with the health sector challenges in the next two decades.

PLAN INDIA

I joined Plan India, an NGO working on women and child health and rights issues, as a Board member in 2016. It is an engaging Board ably chaired by my IAS colleague and long-time friend Rathi Vinay Jha. The key areas of work for Plan India included adolescent health, maternal health and child survival, water, sanitation and hygiene, quality education, youth employment, child protection and disaster-risk management.

Plan India is also a recipient of Global Fund grant for implementation of a programme AHANA for prevention of mother-to-child transmission of HIV in 14 states covering 357 districts with an investment of $16.6 million. The specific goal is to promote periphery-level HIV screening among pregnant women as part of antenatal care (ANC) for early identification of positive pregnant women and linking them with prevention of mother-to-child transmission (PMTCT) services. From October 2015 till date it has reached 28 million pregnant women who had taken an HIV test and about 10,000 among them were found positive and linked to antiretroviral therapy (ART) services. Only 230 infants were found HIV-positive among them, showing the low infectivity rate in the project states. I suggested constitution of a technical advisory committee to provide inputs for efficient management of the grant. The periodic field visits arranged by the secretariat for the Board members were very educative and bore testimony to the impact the programmes were making on peoples' lives.

SWASTI

I was invited to join the Board of Swasti, an International Health Resource Centre established in 2002 in Bangalore by a group of committed public health experts. The objective was to enhance the health and well-being of communities, particularly the marginalised. Swasti's main focus lies in the areas of primary health, sexual and reproductive health including HIV, communicable and noncommunicable diseases, water, sanitation and hygiene and gender-based violence. Shivkumar, one of the cofounders, and Angela Chaudhuri wanted me to join -the Board of Management and share my experience of working in public health programmes including HIV/ AIDS. I knew them and the work they were doing and had no hesitation in joining the Board.

HIGH-LEVEL COMMITTEES OF NACO

After my retirement from the Government of India in December 2004, my contact with the national AIDS programme remained very remote. I visited NACO a few times as part of UNAIDS missions or on a courtesy call. But as I was winding up my commitments as Special Envoy of UNSG, I was called upon by the government to chair in quick succession, three important committees constituted by NACO to bring in governance reforms in the organisation. In February 2016, DG NACO, Navreet Kang, asked me to chair the Mid-Term Review Committee for NACP IV. I had to regret as I was about to go on a 4-month vacation to United States to spend time with my children. The review was completed by the time I returned. Kang wanted me to take the review process forward by chairing a high-level committee (HLC) on consolidation of AIDS response based on the mid-term review and repositioning of NACO to meet new challenges.

HIGH-LEVEL COMMITTEE ON SUSTAINED AIDS RESPONSE

In September 2016, a 10-member HLC was constituted with me as chair to recommend on how to sustain AIDS response and shift gears to achieve the targets set for 2020 in order to meet the goal of ending AIDS by 2030 and how to bring AIDS out of isolation by selective integration of the biomedical services with the health systems and focus more on prevention and allied issues which are exceptional to AIDS.

We held two sittings of the Committee in September and October 2016 and sent our recommendations to DG NACO and Health Secretary. (*Report of HLC, October 2016.*)

Apart from programmatic issues, we specifically suggested important governance reforms in NACO and health ministry to bring synergy in programme management. We suggested that tuberculosis (TB), hepatitis C and drug de-addiction programmes should be brought under the management of NACO and blood safety should be handled by the National Health Mission (NHM) as a general health system issue. The state AIDS control societies need to be remodeled to take care of new demands. The National AIDS Committee (NAC) should be reconstituted as a lean and efficient body which can meet more frequently and provide policy directions to the national programme.

One important outcome of our recommendations was the decision of government to bring in TB programmes under DG NACO to implement the PM's policy directive making TB elimination a national priority to be accomplished by 2025 in India.

However, there was an immediate setback. Navreet Kang who was trying to stabilise the rocking boat of NACO was suddenly moved out in November 2016 along with his joint secretary. This unexpected development had thrown us all off-gear. We could not understand what to make out of it. An additional secretary of health ministry was asked to hold charge and suddenly everything became quiet! It proved very difficult to organise any follow-up with NACO for either UNAIDS or the civil society who welcomed the HLC report as positive.

COMMITTEE OF EXPERTS ON RULES FOR HIV/AIDS ACT

After a period of uncertainty and quick rotation of top officials, Sanjeeva Kumar, the new DG took charge in 2017. He was keen to infuse new dynamism into the national programme which was witnessing frequent changes of leadership in NACO. He was keen to see that the HIV/AIDS Act enacted by the Indian Government in April 2017 was taken up for implementation without delay. He asked me to head a Committee of Experts (CoE) to frame rules and regulations which had to be notified by the Government of India and various state governments to bring the provisions of the Act into effect.

I was happy to get this opportunity to revisit the Act which saw the light of the day after several years of effort. The Act was first contemplated in 2002 when I was heading NACO and had a chequered history. It went through multiple iterations and did several rounds between NACO, Health Ministry and Law Ministry. Three governments had changed in between before the Act could be considered and approved by the Indian Parliament. The President of India finally gave his assent to the legislation in April 2017. There was great excitement among civil society representatives that the Act could finally see the light of the day. Under its provisions, the Act comes into effect only after Rules and Regulations were framed and notified by the central and state governments. Sanjeeva Kumar wanted early enforcement of the provisions of the Act and wanted a quick report from the Committee to facilitate this process.

We held our first meeting in December 2017 and considered the terms of reference. Six major components of the HIV/AIDS Act 2017 were presented before the Committee: (1) address stigma and discrimination, (2) provide an enabling environment for enhancing access to services, (3) safeguard rights of patients living with HIV (PLHIV) and those affected by HIV, (4) provide free diagnostic facilities related to antiretroviral therapies (ARTs), (5) promote safe workplace in health care settings to prevent occupational exposure and (6) strengthen system of grievance redressal. We realised at the outset that the Act was meant to provide necessary protection to only people living with HIV/AIDS and did not cover noninfected persons from the LGBTQ community and people who use drugs.

As the Act was of vital concern to the civil society specially the PLHA population, we decided to secure their involvement by holding regional consultations in north, south and northeastern regions. They were all done back to back in December 2017 itself with tremendous support from the NACO team. The CoE also formed three subcommittees to deliberate on thematic areas namely Ombudsman, HIV/AIDS Policy in Establishments and harmonisation of various guidelines issued by NACO from time to time. The subcommittees met on various dates in January 2018. The CoE met the second and last time in February 2018, finalised its recommendations and sent the draft rules to DG NACO for getting vetted by Law Ministry and promulgation.

Sanjeeva Kumar and his team did a marvelous job in getting all the necessary clearances and promulgated the rules in September 2018, finally bringing the HIV/AIDS Act into force. It was a promise we made to civil society in 2002 but could finally redeem it 16 years later!

HIGH-LEVEL COMMITTEE FOR CONVERGENCE OF AIDS AND TB PROGRAMMES

In March 2018, a month after the CoE submitted its report on rule framing for the HIV/AIDS Act, the Ministry of Health and Family Welfare took an important policy decision to bring the Revised National TB Control Programme (RNTCP) under the control of DG NACO by designating him as DG RNTCP and placing the Central TB Division under his charge. RNTCP would follow the same organisational structure and channels of submission already prevalent in NACO to bring in synergies for fast tracking both the programmes as envisaged in the National Health Policy 2017. This order was a follow-up to the PM Narendra Modi's policy initiative to prioritise TB elimination in India by advancing the target date by 5 years to 2025.

In April 2018, Sanjeeva Kumar decided to constitute an HLC for suggesting measures for better management of the two national programmes at national, state and district levels and to develop strategies and convergence in implementation between the two programmes by adopting a patient-centric approach. I was asked to chair this committee also. Two former secretaries from the Health Ministry, Deepak Gupta and V.M. Katoch were also invited to join along with six other members.

We had our first meeting in May 2018 and identified three broad areas of convergence between the two programmes (1) the governance structures at centre, state and district levels, (2) service delivery mechanisms of both programmes and (3) involvement of civil society and private sector. Three subgroups were asked to deliberate on these areas and report back to the main committee. After receipt of the reports from the three subgroups, the HLC met a final time in June 2018 and adopted its recommendations.

We were aware that convergence of two large disease control programmes needs to be done with due care and diligence. The AIDS control programme is a central sector programme with full funding from the Government of India while the TB programme is a centrally sponsored programme with sharing of funds between centre and the states. If true convergence had to be brought in, it is necessary to bring in uniformity of funding for both programmes and adopt the same method of fund transfers at state and district levels. Governance structures at centre and state level need to be integrated as a follow-up measure to the designation of DG NACO as DG RNTCP.

For service delivery, we felt that the distinct characteristics of the two programmes had to be retained and co-location of facilities and sharing of technical personnel should be explored to bring in optimisation. Civil society engagement which was a distinct feature of AIDS programme should be adopted with modifications for the TB programme as well.

We also reiterated the recommendations of the earlier HLC on integration of services that blood safety should be merged with NHM and hepatitis C and drug de-addiction programmes should be brought under NACO.

The report was sent to DG NACO/RNTCP and the Health Secretary in July 2018.

Quite unexpectedly, the recommendations did not find favour with the officials of National Health Mission (NHM), especially those relating to control of TB budget which currently lies with NHM. If effective convergence had to take place the DG who is tasked to run both programmes should have control over the availability and release of funds as part of the budgetary mechanism. In a meeting called by the Health Secretary on 31 July 2018, the NHM officials from centre and the states vehemently opposed the convergence idea. Sanjeeva Kumar who was holding both the charges as DG expressed clearly that he will be greatly handicapped if he had no control on the TB budget and had to knock at the doors of NHM every time he needed release of funds. I could see that within the ministry there was no unanimity on the convergence idea despite the PM's directive. The health secretary at the end wanted to bring the matter to the minister's attention as two senior officials of the ministry were having divergent views.

I was very disappointed that the government was missing an excellent opportunity of implementing a convergence model for two large public health programmes which could later be adopted to bring in other programmes for control of communicable and noncommunicable diseases under a single governance structure. The health ministry had become too large and cumbersome to handle diverse nature of work, partly regulatory and partly developmental. Reform of its governance structure is overdue. Carving out a separate department of public health to take care of all the public health programmes would relieve the burden from the main department of health which can focus more on policy, coordination and regulatory issues. Constitution of a separate cadre of public health professionals at central and state level would have fitted very well with this bifurcated structure of health ministry.

Experience of past 20 years has shown that health sector in India and many developing countries still remains underfunded and the weakness of public health care infrastructure gets repeatedly exposed with onslaught of one or the other epidemics–latest being the Covid19 pandemic. A carefully thought out reorganization of health sector is overdue both in Government of India and the states.

EPILOGUE

For 20 years, working on AIDS campaigns as part of the health sector, the bitter truth I've learnt is that although the health of a nation is inextricably linked with the health of its people, this comes very low in national priorities. Health, these days, is synonymous with health care, that is, hospitals and institutions, with a provider-centric focus, while a truly people-centric approach only exists in policy documentation. This can be attributed to the long gestation period before public health programmes such as health promotion, nutrition and hygiene truly pay off, leading to disinterest from leaders in developing countries, who opt more for short-term visible gains. Elections are, after all, seldom fought over which party would do better at sanitation, hygiene and nutrition. This leads to a gap between precept and practice and a shift from 'Creating health' to 'Providing healthcare'.

I have witnessed from my own experience that health programmes get fast-tracked when there is political support. As a member of the civil service in India, I often thought that efficient implementation of programmes can be secured by administrative ability and commitment. I realised during my journey how much difference enlightened and far-sighted political leadership can make in driving social agendas such as control of HIV/AIDS or promotion of public and preventive health. My emphasis in all my country missions was to engage with political leadership and sensitise them about the pitfalls of declining political support for programmes. It is leadership which makes a difference between an ordinary and exceptional response.

A key lesson I learnt while working on HIV/AIDS was the value of good data and information to influence political thinking. Right from my earlier days in NACO I attached great importance to collection and analysis of primary data from the field and use it for political advocacy. I recorded on more than one occasion in this book on how information, when strategically used, can alter the course of response by capturing the attention of those who can do the most good. It is good science and good epidemiology which should inform health sector responses and building institutes of excellence which promote such learning should always remain a political priority.

A whole new world opened before me in working closely with populations who are living on the margins of society with endless stigma facing them. Every visit to a sex worker site or a methadone clinic or an MSM network enhanced my understanding of societal relations from a new and wide-angled lens. I emerged as a much changed and more understanding individual in my work environment and personal life, overcoming many of the prejudices one carries as just another member of mainstream society.

The success of global AIDS response is owed in large measure to a synergistic combination of these broad determinants of public health; a strong and committed leadership willing to provide resources to scale, a strong evidence base built by quality data and information provided by scientific investigation and a vibrant civil society with intimate involvement of communities who are at the centre of the epidemic. And the steady dilution of efforts on all these three fronts in the past few years has brought the global response to its present critical phase.

Viewed in this background, the overall AIDS response in India and at regional and global level continues to cause concern for many of us who have been involved with the AIDS movement since the 1990s. On the positive side, the programme has successfully reduced the spread of the epidemic in many countries in Asia Pacific, Africa, Latin American and Caribbean regions. Exceptions to this general trend are countries such as Indonesia, the Philippines and Pakistan in Asia, which still witness rising number of new infections. Two important regions still showing a rising incidence of HIV are Eastern Europe and Central Asia (EECA) and the Middle East and Northern Africa (MENA). The UNAIDS Global Report 2020 comes with this candid admission.

'Increases in resources for HIV responses in low- and middle-income countries stalled in 2017, and funding decreased by 7% between 2017 and 2019.1 The total HIV funding available in these countries in 2019 amounted to about 70% of the 2020 target set by the UN General Assembly....... This collective failure to invest sufficiently in comprehensive, rights-based HIV responses comes at a terrible price: from 2015 to 2020, there were 3.5 million more HIV infections and 820 000 more AIDS-related deaths than if the world was on track to meet its 2020 targets. The blueprint for success is widely available. The world can do better'.

The Asia Pacific scenario is even more glaring. An overwhelming 98% of new infections have occurred among key populations and their partners. New infections dropped only by 12% in the past 10 years working out to an average of 1.2% per year which is statistically insignificant.

At this rate it is highly doubtful if any country would be able to reach the stiff targets set for 2020 by the high-level meeting (HLM) on AIDS in 2016. For most of them AIDS was no longer a priority public health concern. A stock taking which might occur in 2021 would expose this collective failure of member nations in honouring their commitment on AIDS made just 4 years ago.

This is a critical time when UNAIDS, the Joint UN programme should have been the leading player for global advocacy on AIDS. But the organisation itself had run into serious internal crisis in 2018 with a senior-level professional in Geneva leaving the organisation on sexual harassment charges. An independent assessment ordered by the PCB on the state of affairs prevailing in UNAIDS gave a damaging report on the working conditions of women staff. The Executive Director, Michel Sidibe, announced in a PCB meeting that he would leave the organisation in 2019 after the June meeting. He was later appointed as the Health Minister, Mali, and left earlier than the scheduled date. The new Executive Director, Winnie Byanyima, assumed the reins of office in August 2019 and expressed her strong intent to improve the quality of workplace for women in the organisation. Byanyima was the Executive Director of Oxfam International since 2013 and prior to that, served for 7 years as the Director of Gender and Development at the UNDP. It will involve a substantial amount of effort from her to restore the credibility of UNAIDS to regain its unique position as a leading global advocate for AIDS.

In an opinion piece in the national newspaper *The Hindu,* I tried to identify three major strategic issues which need attention from the UNAIDS top management. First was the highly positive messaging of the past few years from UNAIDS that the world was going to see the end of AIDS very soon. These campaigns resulted in complacency among political leadership in the countries. Second was the thinking that AIDS epidemic can simply be treated away by saturating ART coverage among infected populations. In the process, prevention programmes took a back seat in high prevalence countries which proved costly. Third was the weakening of UNAIDS country leadership in high prevalence countries which was more an issue of internal governance within the organisation. I pleaded for a re-energised UNAIDS with a strong and fearless leadership capable of taking difficult decisions. In order to make an impact, the new executive director should address these priority challenges.

A promising development in this otherwise gloomy scenario was the commitment made by the international donor community to the GFATM for funding the Global AIDS, TB and Malaria programmes. Donors at the Global Fund's Sixth Replenishment Conference in 2019 pledged $14.02 billion for the next 3 years–the largest amount ever raised for a multilateral health organisation, and the largest amount by the Global Fund. The funds are expected to save 16 million lives and end the epidemics of AIDS, TB and malaria by 2030.

An important target set for countries for 2020 was the elimination of mother-to-child transmission (eMTCT). It is heartening to see that many countries are on their way to achieve this important landmark. In Asia region, Thailand, Sri Lanka and Maldives have already declared eMTCT in the past 2 years. Other countries should get inspired by this performance and follow suit.

But it is in the area prevention that countries encounter their toughest challenge. New technologies such as pre-exposure prophylaxis (PrEP) have been successfully pilot tested and included in the national response in Australia and Thailand. PrEP offers lot of hope for vulnerable communities namely men who have sex with men (MSM) and sex workers for protecting themselves from HIV. The Global Coalition on Prevention which was set up in the aftermath of the HLM 2016 could not garner critical political support to function as an effective advocacy group on prevention. UNAIDS needs to focus its efforts on rejuvenating the Coalition, supported by a strong group of technical experts on prevention assembled in its Headquarters in Geneva. Substantial part of the new funds from GFATM should flow to prevention programmes in high prevalence countries to bring down new infections to the targeted level in the next 2 to 3 years.

Much of the above applies to India's AIDS response too. Prevention and treatment programmes have to be fully funded based on unit costs of interventions. NACP IV was consistently getting lesser resources in the budget than what were projected under the approved scheme. Its extension up to 2020 without commitment of additional funds has constrained its resource base to the existing level. Time is ripe to plan for phase V of NACP with clearly identifiable targets and full funding based on unit costs of intervention. The states which are in the forefront of implementation of programmes have a critical role to play in getting AIDS back into the political discourse. Senior and committed officials should be deployed full time at leadership levels to manage the programme. Civil society voices that have become mute in the past few years need to be heard again. Monitoring and supervision of programmes has greatly suffered in the past few years as AIDS became a part-time job for many project directors at the state level. The strong bond that existed earlier between NACO and state AIDS control societies and civil society needs to be restored to make the programme truly participatory. Senior-level functionaries with civil society background and experience should be inducted into NACO to take charge of programmes that have a civil society interface. Specific recommendations made in the aide memoire we submitted to the government at the end of the UNAIDS mission in 2017 are very relevant at this moment.

The road to elimination of AIDS as a public health threat will not be easy. I stand by what I said at the last PCB of UNAIDS in June 2017. 'Please tell the world that AIDS is not over! Not yet. And countries which have set for themselves the task of ending AIDS by 2030 should not rest until it is over'.

The world still has a window of opportunity to close the gap between the goals and achievements to end AIDS as a public health concern. There will be successes and failures on the way but a sense of optimism and positive thinking should pervade the AIDS response. We should learn to celebrate small victories but take lessons from failures to march ahead. On that optimistic note I end this narrative.

INDEX

Printed in Great Britain
by Amazon

55083838R00166